Edited by
DINESH BHUGRA
and **VEENA BAHL**

DATE DUE

Ethr
for]

GASKELL

© The Royal College of Psychiatrists 1999.

Gaskell is an imprint of the Royal College of Psychiatrists
17 Belgrave Square, London SW1X 8PG

British Library Cataloguing-in-Publication Data
A catalogue record for this book is available from the British Library.
ISBN 1-901242-15-3

Distributed in North America
by American Psychiatric Press, Inc.
ISBN 0-88048-585-X

Cover design by Graphic Creative, West Sussex
Printed by Bell & Bain Ltd, Glasgow

Contents

Contributors

Melanie Abas, Institute of Psychiatry, De Crespigny Park, London SE5 8AF

Veena Bahl, Department of Health, Wellington House, 133–155 Waterloo Road, London SE1 8UG

David Baldwin, University of Southampton, Department of Psychiatry, Royal South Hampshire Hospital, Graham Road, Southampton, Hants SO9 4PE

Dinesh Bhugra, Institute of Psychiatry, De Crespigny Park, London SE5 8AF

Kamaldeep Bhui, Institute of Psychiatry, De Crespigny Park, London SE5 8AF

Raymond Cochrane, School of Psychology, University of Birmingham, Edgbaston, Birmingham, B15 2TT

Eleanor Cole, Maudsley Hospital, Denmark Hill, London SE5 8AF

Julia Deane, Projecto Saude e al Algegia, TV Dom Anando 697, Santeren-PA 68005–420, Brazil

Manisha Desai, Institute of Psychiatry, De Crespigny Park, London SE5 8AF

Peter Gluckman, Lambeth, Southwark and Lewisham Purchasing Authority, 1 Lower Marsh, London SE1 7NT

David Goldberg, Institute of Psychiatry, De Crespigny Park, London SE5 8AF

Carol M. Grant-Pearce, PREST, University of Manchester, Oxford Road, Manchester M13 9PL

Pat Gray, Barnado's Family Service, Mornington Terrace, Liverpool, L1 9DY

Richard Hackett, Holly House, Gladstone Terrace Road, Greenfield, Oldham, OL3 7HF

N. Kibe, The Tavistock Centre, London

R. Kumar, Perinatal Section, Institute of Psychiatry, De Crespigny Park, London SE5 8AF

Janet La Grenade, Department of Community Health & Psychiatry, University of West Indies, Mona Campus, Kingston 7, Jamaica

Sunjai Gupta, Department of Health, Wellington House, 133–155 Waterloo Road, London SE1 8UG

Julian Leff, MRC Social Genetic and Development Centre, Institute of Psychiatry, De Crespigny Park, London SE5 8AF

Rachael Lippett, Institute of Psychiatry, De Crespigny Park, London SE5 8AF

Keith Lloyd, Department of Mental Health, University of Exeter, Wonford House Hospital, Exeter EX2 5AF

Kwame McKenzie, Institute of Psychiatry, De Crespigny Park, London SE5 8AF

Tony Maden, Institute of Psychiatry, De Crespigny Park, London SE5 8AF

Maureen N. Marks, Perinatal Section, Institute of Psychiatry, De Crespigny Park, London SE5 8AF

A. Matsumoto, Department of Neuropsychiatry, Faculty of Medicine, Kyushu University, Fukuoka, Japan

Robin M. Murray, Institute of Psychiatry, De Crespigny Park, London SE5 8AF

H. Nakano, Department of Obstetrics and Gynaecology, Faculty of Medicine, Kyushu University, Fukuoka, Japan

Sue Parkman, PRiSM, Institute of Psychiatry, De Crespigny Park, London SE5 8AF

Sangeeta Patel, St George's Hospital Medical School, Division of General Practice and Primary Care, Hunter Wing, Cranmer Terrace, London SW17 0RE

Marcus Richards, Institute of Psychiatry, De Crespigny Park, London SE5 8AF

Mirelia Ruggeri, Department of Psychological Medicine, Ospedale Policlinico, 37134 Verona, Italy

Lynn St Louis, Institute of Psychiatry, De Crespigny Park, London SE5 8AF

S. P. Sashidharan, North Birmingham Mental Health Trust, Academic Unit, 71 Fentham Road, Erdingham, Birmingham B23 6AL

N. Tashiro, Department of Neuropsychiatry, Faculty of Medicine, Kyushu University, Fukuoka, Japan

Graham Thornicroft, PRiSM, Institute of Psychiatry, De Crespigny Park, London SE5 8AF

Indira Vyas, Child & Family Psychiatric Service, Westcotes House, Westcotes Drive, Leicester LE3 0QU

H. Yamashita, Department of Neuropsychiatry, Faculty of Medicine, Kyushu University, Fukuoka, Japan

K. Yoshida, Perinatal Section, Institute of Psychiatry, University of London

Foreword

The report *Modernising Mental Health Services* (Department of Health, 1998) sets out the Government's vision for safe, sound and supportive mental health services. *Our Healthier Nation* (Secretary of State, 1998) sets out the Government's agenda for tackling inequalities in health. It is clear that modern mental health services should be evidence-based, recognise the differing needs of the diverse community groups in the population and provide care which is integrated.

It is well known that Black and minority ethnic groups find it difficult to access mental health services through primary care and there are high rates of certain mental illnesses in some Black and minority ethnic groups. The nature of mental illness in relation to Black and minority ethnic groups is not always understood by health and social services and requires continuous assessment and an improved knowledge base.

Both the Green Paper *Our Healthier Nation* and the *Inequalities in Health* report (Acheson, 1998) provide a new opportunity to address mental health of Black and minority ethnic groups and offers an approach to tackling mental health of Black and minority ethnic groups based on local intiatives.

References

ACHESON, D. (1998) *Independent Inquiry into Inequalities in Health Report.* London: HMSO.
DEPARTMENT OF HEALTH (1998) *Modernising Mental Health Services: Safe, Sound and Supportive.* London: Department of Health.
SECRETARY OF STATE (1998*b*) *Our Healthier Nation.* London: HMSO.

Tessa Jowell, MP
Minister for Public Health
Department of Health

Preface

DINESH BHUGRA and VEENA BAHL

Mental health is a subject which has been of relevance and importance to governments as well as Black and ethnic groups for a number
of years for a number of reasons. There remain key issues in delivery
of mental health services which have highlighted serious gaps in
provision in various parts, yet at the same time there are examples
of good clinical practice which deserve better exposure. Some of
the key topics in delivery in mental health services as well as clinical
research have been the over-representation of African–Caribbean
patients in hospital, being treated with more physical therapies and
being diagnosed as having schizophrenia. Several studies have
suggested that schizophrenia is indeed more common in African–
Caribbean groups, whereas for South Asians attempted suicide in
women and problems of alcohol misuse in men are higher than the
native population. The health needs of minority ethnic groups and
Black patients vary. The recent White Papers on the future of the
National Health Service (NHS) for England, Wales and Scotland,
along with the Green Paper *Our Healthier Nation*, provide a framework
within which service delivery can be improved. With an emphasis
on Primary Care Services it is important that psychiatrists and other
mental health professionals take into account the needs of Black
and minority ethnic groups. These proposed changes in the delivery
of services within the NHS provide a suitable opportunity for
involving the stakeholders at local level and also giving the
communities a voice. With the problems of social exclusion linked
intimately with the mental health needs of Black and minority ethnic
groups it is essential that the service providers are aware of the
problems in delivery as well as acceptance of clinical services as they
stand. Voluntary organisations have often been more successful than
statutory services by involving the communities at a very local level
in planning and delivery of services and taking into account their
opinions and views about the models of illness as well as requirements from services. These changes are an essential element in

bringing about the change in the delivery of mental health services and also involving voluntary organisations at a much closer level than has been done hitherto.

In 1995 the Department of Health funded a two-day, closed, round-table conference on the role of ethnicity and culture in mental health. This conference was attended by epidemiologists, researchers, clinicians, purchasers as well as representatives from voluntary organisations who contributed to the discussions. This book is a compilation of the discussions that went on at the conference. In addition, we have commissioned some special chapters to add to the discussion and take the agenda of service delivery for Black and minority ethnic groups forward. We are grateful to the Department of Health for funding the conference and for the publication of this book.

1 Ethnicity – issues of definition

DINESH BHUGRA and VEENA BAHL

Ethnicity, ethnic identity or ethnic group are terms used to describe a characteristic which may 'identify' an individual to others. It is like describing a person or even oneself while writing to a distant pen-friend for the first time. One would like to develop and maintain watertight definitions for ethnicity, but neat boundaries and operational criteria are not always possible. There is no doubt that ethnicity, ethnic identity and ethnic group all point towards a set of cognitive schemata and behaviours which may shape the functioning of the individual at one level and of the family, society or culture at another. This consistency of behaviour can be deemed to be a non-changing, non-influenced characteristic – although we may find that it is not always very clear.

Royce (1982) proposes that ethnicity can be approached in two ways: the first is a neo-Marxist approach characterising studies of ethnicity and identity primarily at an institutional level. The second is the psychoanalytic approach, which focuses on the individual. The basic argument is that the neo-Marxist approach ignores the problems of ethnic minorities within their boundaries, as demonstrated in the Soviet Union and China. These problems have been related to social class. Such an approach has little empirical value in most of the situations of ethnic interaction in the contemporary world.

In the USA, ethnic groups are said to be:

"characterised by some of the following features: common geographic origins; migratory status; race; language or dialect; religions, faith or faiths; ties transcending kinship neighbourhood and community boundaries; shared traditions; values and symbols; literature; folklore and music; food preferences; settlement and employment patterns; special interest in regard to politics in the homeland and in the US; institutions that specifically serve and maintain the group; an internal sense of distinctiveness and an external perception of distinctiveness" (Thernstrom *et al*, 1980).

This series of characteristics lacks any rigour and appears to be most inclusive. It is difficult to know how many of these characteristics are essential, and how many are desirable. Smith (1993) includes the most extensive definition, but ignores the explicit requirement of whether or not all of the 14 characteristics distinguish all groups or all members of an ethnic group at any level of intensity, separately or together. Smith (1993) goes on to argue that when authors treat 'race' as one criterion of ethnicity then inter-racial relationships therefore must be seen as 'different' according to the existing definitions.

Associated factors

McKenzie & Crowcroft (1996) observe that with changes in fashion, terms change and clinicians must be aware of underlying issues. Royce (1982) suggests that three factors are associated with ethnic identity – power, perception and purpose. The first of these factors, power, is perhaps primary. This imposition of power on individuals can affect other definitions, and other considerations including perception and purpose then become secondary. Thus Royce (1982) argues that, bearing in mind this proposition, one corollary is that everyone in a subordinate position is potentially a member of an ethnic group and the dominant group has the privilege to assign roles and lay down rules. By definition, dominant individuals are likely to have more power that subordinates – the power stems from having historical, material and ideological resources. On this principle, at least one study demonstrated that Black students were more aware than the White students were of themselves – the Black students saw themselves and were conscious of their minority status, but the White students did not see themselves as distinctly White (Szalazay & Deese, 1978).

Contemporary relationships between various ethnic groups and the dominant powers have to be seen in their historical context. Politics in most post-independence, less-developed countries are linked with one ethnic group dominating others. Such a multi-ethnic mosaic was itself a creation of colonialism (Premdas, 1993). The pillars used for such a model according to Premdas (1993) were: dependence (largely economic), centralisation, discrimination, co-optation, segmentation, terror and manipulation of ethnic symbols.

Smith (1993) points out that in recent times race as a concept has been defined in relation to colonial factors (i.e. historical forces) along with political interpretations. The potent combination of emerging new countries with specific national identities and nationalism along with changing power patterns was bound to ignite emotions which further complicate any attempts at definitions. Traditional concepts of race have had their own difficulties. It was suggested that each of the phenotypically distinct races had a distinct set of psychological attributes and cultural potentials and that entire populations could be assigned to one or other of a limited number of racial stocks. These subdivisions were 'fixed' and there existed a natural hierarchy (Biddiss, 1970). This process of 'racism', where one body of thought holds some ethnic groups as superior or inferior to others on hereditary grounds (precluding prospects of change), does affect the definitions and acceptance of certain ethnic identities. Smith (1993) goes on to define racialism as the institutional practice and structure of domination and discrimination or preference on the basis of differentiating people on racial grounds (Benedict, 1943; Van den Berghe, 1967; Rex, 1970; also see Chapters 20 and 21). Often this distinction between racism and racialism is forgotten by academics and laymen alike.

Definitions

We have drawn attention to 14 characteristics of ethnic identity, following Royce's (1982) pointer that ethnic was defined as:

> "neither Christian nor Jewish; heathen; of or relating to races or large groups of people classed according to common traits or customs" (Webster's 7th Collegiate Dictionary).

She stresses that such definitions provide the basis from which most people derive their ideas about appropriate attitudes and behaviour towards others. Isajiw (1974) listed 12 characteristics, of which the most common five were: common ancestral origin, same culture or customs, religion, race or physical characteristics and language. These attributes are immediately apparent and easily checked. The others included many characteristics based on feelings of status, common values or ethos and relations. Such a definition, therefore, especially based on the first five characteristics, is an objective definition. Senior & Bhopal (1994) urge that ethnicity should be differentiated from race. Furthermore, ethnicity is not a sound epidemiological variable because of problems of definition, problems of heterogeneity in the population and ethnocentricity among researchers, among other factors. They highlight some of the studies which focus on pathology in ethnic minorities rather than attempting to understand communities.

Despite the difficulties of definition a recent inspection of community care services for Black and ethnic minority older people has led to the following definitions.

(a) Ethnic minority: relates to all subgroups of the population not indigenous to the UK who hold cultural traditions and values derived, at least in part, from their countries of origin. This therefore excludes national minorities such as the Scottish, Northern Irish and Welsh, but they equally have the right to have their distinctive cultural traditions and values respected in the way that they are offered services.

(b) Black: refers to those members of ethnic minority groups who are differentiated by their skin colour or physical appearance, and may therefore feel some solidarity with one another by reason of past or current experience, but who may have many different cultural traditions and values.

Self-concept and self-ascription

On the other hand, subjective definitions are the definitions that individuals ascribe to themselves. They may identify themselves as being different from others or belonging to a different group. They may be identified as being different by others. This is a mixture of both self and other ascriptions (Royce, 1982). There are also the possibilities of composite definitions as follows:

"... any group which is defined or set off by race, religion or national origin or some combination of these categories" (Gordon, 1964).

Shibutani & Kwan (1965) define ethnic groups as:

"... people who conceive of themselves as being of a kind. They are united by emotional bonds and conceived with the preservation of their type. With very few exceptions, they speak the same language, or their speech is at least intelligible to each other and they share a common cultural heritage. Since those who form such units are usually endogamous, they tend to look alike. Far more important, however, is their belief that they are of common descent, a belief usually supported by myths or a partly fictitious history".

The Office of Population Censuses and Surveys' (OPCS) introduction of ethnic identity in the British census data collection relies on subjective definition. There are, of course, problems with such categorisation – the features of identity may change without changing the self-identity and *vice versa*. The differential rate of change of objective states remains a valuable area of research. Contemporary definitions on the other hand include different criteria. The Social Sciences Research Council (SSRC, 1974) identified six criteria for the definition of ethnicity: a past-oriented group identification emphasising origins; some conceptions of cultural and social distinctiveness; relationship of the ethnic group to a component unit in a broader system of social relations; the fact that ethnic groups are larger than kin or locality groups and transcend face-to-face interaction; different meanings for ethnic categories both in different social settings and for different individuals; and the assumption that ethnic categories are emblematic, having names with meaning both for members and analysts. Royce (1982) argues that the SSRC definition is unwieldy, and she offers a succinct alternative:

"... an ethnic group is a reference group invoked by people who share a common historical style (which may only be assumed), based on overt features and values, and who, through the process of interaction with others, identify themselves as sharing that style".

De Vos (1975) suggests that the ethnic identity, like any form of identity, is not only a question of knowing who one is subjectively, but also of how one is seen from the outside: "Ethnic identity requires the maintenance of sufficiently consistent behaviour to enable others to place an individual or a group in some given social category". Thus, to summarise Royce (1982), definitions of ethnicity or ethnic identity must be composed of both subjective and objective components and support the notion that ethnic groups are eminently mutable, providing another reference group with which individuals can vary their social strategies.

Although McKenzie & Crowcroft (1994) suggest that terminology must reflect the hypothesis under consideration, this is a difficult recommendation to follow, and would make comparisons across different ethnic groups in different cultures virtually impossible. However, defined groups should be adequately described in the research dissemination. This may well be in addition to self-ascription (McKenzie & Crowcroft, 1996). Any definition of ethnicity remains a difficult area. There needs to be a uniformity in purpose and national or international agreements need to be reached.

References

BENEDICT, R. (1943) *Race, Science and Politics*. New York: Viking.

BIDDISS, M. D. (1970) *Father of Racist Idealogy*. London: Jonathan Cape.

DE VOS, G. (1975) Ethnic pluralism. In *Ethnic Identity: Cultural Continuities and Change* (eds I. G. De Vos & L. Romanucci-Ross). Palo Alto, CA: Mayfield.

GORDON, M. (1964) *Assimilation in American Life: the Role of Race, Religion and National Origins*. New York: Open University Press.

ISAJIW, W. (1974) Definitions of ethnicity. *Ethnicity*, 1, 111–124.

McKenzie, K. & Crowcroft, N. (1994) Race, ethnicity, culture and science. *British Medical Journal*, **309**, 286–287.

—— & —— (1996) Describing race, ethnicity and culture in medical research. *British Medical Journal*, **312**, 1054.

Premdas, R. P. (1993) The anatomy of ethnic conflict: domination *versus* reconciliation. In *The Enigma of Ethnicity: An Analysis of Race in the Caribbean and the World* (ed. R. Premdas). St Augustine, Trinidad: UWI Press.

Rex, J. (1970) *Race Relations in Sociological Theory*. London: Weidenfeld and Nicholson.

Royce, A. P. (1982) *Ethnic Identity: Strategies of Diversity*. Bloomington, IA: Indiana University Press.

Senior, P. & Bhopal, R. (1994) Ethnicity in health research. *British Medical Journal*, **309**, 327–330.

Shibutani, T. & Kwan, K. M. (1965) *Ethnic Stratification*. New York: Macmillan.

Smith, M. G. (1993) Race and ethnicity. In *The Enigma of Ethnicity: An Analysis of Race in the Caribbean and the World* (ed. R. Premdas). St Augustine, Trinidad: UWI Press.

SSRC (1974) *Comparative Research on Ethnicity: A Conference Report* (ed. W. Bell). New York: SSRC.

Szalazay, L. B. & Deese, J. E. (1978) *Selective Meaning and Culture: An Assessment Through Word Association*. New York: Halstead Press.

Thernstrom, S., Orlov, A. & Handlin, O. (eds) (1980) *The Harvard Encyclopedia of American Ethnic Groups*. Cambridge, MA: Harvard University Press.

Van den Berghe, P. (1967) *Race and Racism: A Comparative Perspective*. New York: John Wiley and Sons.

2 Mental illness: a national perspective

VEENA BAHL

Mental illness is a subject which has been discussed for a number of years in the context of ethnic minority health both by the community and psychiatrists. A range of explanations about the increased rates of certain types of mental illness among ethnic minority groups in Britain has been put forward by both groups. The explanations point towards the need for a better understanding of the issues and a need to improve the mental health of the population and provide appropriate, culturally competent services.

The White Paper *The New NHS: Modern and Dependable* (Secretary of State, 1997), the White Paper *Modernising Social Services* (Secretary of State, 1998*a*) and the Green Paper *Our Healthier Nation* (Secretary of State, 1998*b*) provide an opportunity to examine mental health in the context of providing a seamless approach to health and social care. The report into inequalities in health (Acheson, 1998) sets ethnic minority health within the inequalities in health agenda and provides a focus to tackle the root causes of mental illness and suicide.

The report *Modernising Mental Health Services* (Department of Health, 1998) sets out the Government's vision for the future delivery of mental health services. The 'Mental Health National Service Framework', to be published in the spring of 1999, will set standards and identify service models.

All of the above-cited reports provide a new challenge to address ethnicity and health in a wider context, including social determinants which impact on health such as poverty.

Black and minority ethnic communities form approximately 6% of the population, that is, 3 000 000 people in England and Wales (see Fig. 1). The ethnic groups show marked variations in their geographical distribution across the country and in their level of geographical concentration. Black Caribbean, Black African and

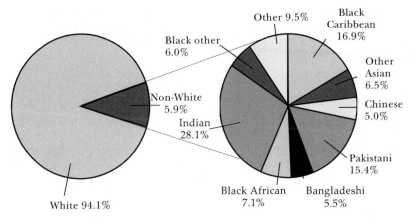

FIG. 1
Ethnic composition of the population of England and Wales

TABLE 1
Decisions on asylum applications in the UK, 1987–1997

	1987	1988	1989	1990	1991	1992	1993	1994	1995	1996	1997
Refugee status											
%	11	23	32	23	10	6	9	5	5	6	13
n	266	628	2210	920	505	1115	1590	825	1295	2240	3985
ELR											
%	63	58	55	60	44	80	64	21	19	14	11
n	1531	1578	3860	2400	2190	15 325	11 125	3360	4410	5055	3115
Refusals											
%	26	19	13	17	46	14	27	74	76	80	76
n	635	496	890	705	2325	2675	4705	12 655	17 705	28 040	22 780

ELR, exceptional leave to remain.
Decision figures exclude refusals made without substantive consideration of the
asylum application as follows. 1992: 15 195 refused under paragraph 101 and 595
refused on safe third country grounds; 1993: 5240 refused under paragraph 180F
and 745 refused on safe third country grounds; 1994: 2985 refused under paragraph
340 and 865 refused on safe third country grounds; 1995: 2085 refused under
paragraph 340 and 1515 refused on safe third country grounds; 1996: 2015 refused
under paragraph 340 and 1615 refused on safe third country grounds; 1997: 3615
refused under paragraph 340 and 2550 refused on safe third country grounds.

Bangladeshi people live predominantly in the Greater London area,
mostly in inner London. One-third of the Indian community lives
in the outer London suburbs, with substantial concentrations in the

West Midlands and Leicestershire. In contrast, people of Pakistani origin live in the West Midlands and West Yorkshire. The Chinese are more evenly dispersed than other ethnic groups (National Institute for Ethnic Studies in Health and Social Policy, 1997).

Another important subgroup of ethnic minorities is the refugee community: although the number in the population is small, they represent a challenge for health and social services. Table 1 gives approximate numbers of refugees recognised and granted asylum in Britain.

It should be remembered that Black and minority ethnic health is part of the wider social exclusion agenda. Social determinants such as overcrowding, unemployment, financial strains/pressures and poor housing make it difficult to lead healthier lives (Secretary of State, 1998*b*). Overcrowding is a major issue among some ethnic minority groups. About 2% of White households are overcrowded

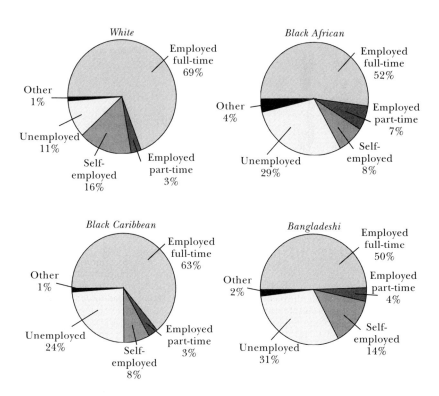

Fɪɢ. 2
Economic status in each ethnic group in England and Wales – economically active males

and 0.3% are severely overcrowded. In contrast almost half (47%) of Bangladeshi households are overcrowded and almost one-fifth (19%)are severely overcrowded. Pakistani households also have higher levels of overcrowding (29%) and severe overcrowding (8%). All other ethnic groups also have higher levels of overcrowding than White households, although not to the same degree as in Bangladeshi and Pakistani households. Unemployment is highest in Bangladeshi men (with about one in three (31%) out of work) and in Pakistani men (29%). About one-quarter of Black African (29%), Black other (26%) and Black Caribbean (24%) people are unemployed (see Fig. 2). In addition, compared with 20% of White households, over one-third (35–41%) of Black households reside in accommodation rented from the local authority or equivalent.

The picture of mental illness is described by Balarajan & Raleigh (1993) and Nazroo (1997) (see also Chapters 5 and 23), who highlight the following facts about mental health.

African–Caribbean population

   (a) African–Caribbean people in Britain have higher admission rates to psychiatric hospitals and are diagnosed as having schizophrenia 3–6 times more often than the White population.

   (b) The incidence of schizophrenia in British-born Caribbean people is proportionately higher than the incidence reported for Jamaica and Trinidad.

   (c) Rates of schizophrenia in second-generation British-born Black people may be greater than the rates in the first generation.

   (d) Black people are over-represented among patients compulsorily detained in psychiatric hospitals under the Mental Health Act, and also through police admissions.

   (e) African–Caribbean people receive differential and stronger forms of treatment, although differences in clinical management can partly be explained by differences in diagnosis.

   (f) Recent research is examining the issue of misdiagnosis among African–Caribbean people.

Asian population

   (a) Some studies show higher hospital admission rates among Asian people than those for the British-born population.

   (b) The balance of evidence from hospital admission rates, general practitioner (GP) consultation rates and community surveys suggests that Asian people have rates of psychiatric morbidity similar to or lower than the indigenous population.

(c) In primary care, rates of depression and anxiety among Asian attendees are comparable with the indigenous population (Nazroo, 1997).

(d) It is not known whether these patterns reflect genuinely lower psychiatric morbidity or differences in detection rates, reluctance of Asian people to present themselves as having mental health problems, or differences in the manner of presentation (see Chapter 23).

(e) Linguistic and/or communication problems make it harder for GPs to recognise such problems when they arise. It is possible, therefore, that there is an element of unrecognised and untreated psychiatric morbidity within this ethnic group, which may be greater than in the indigenous population.

(f) Suicide rates are low in some subgroups born on the Indian subcontinent, whereas women born in India or east Africa show a significant excess (see Chapter 12).

(g) The rate of suicides among first-generation Asian women is greatest among the young. The rate in girls aged 15–24 years who were born on the Indian subcontinent is more than double the national average and at ages 25–34 years is 60% higher in those who were born in India.

(h) Young Asian women also have high rates of attempted suicide, and are clearly a high-risk group in terms of the *Health of the Nation* targets (Department of Health, 1994) for reducing suicide rates.

The social and economic status of Black and minority ethnic groups may influence their mental health status, and this points towards a closer examination of the issues in relation to delivery of services. The following are key issues.

(a) High rates of admissions and readmissions to secondary care of African–Caribbean patients have been a major issue in the past. A recent study (Nazroo, 1997) has shown that the rates may not be as high as has been suggested previously, although this may be for methodological reasons (see Chapter 23). Further research should be done to establish the true incidence rates.

(b) Excessive use of drug therapy for African–Caribbean populations has been shown to be an issue. It is important that health authorities audit treatment and care given to Black and minority ethnic groups.

(c) Quality of services in the medium secure units and recovery rates. It is important that the communities' views of care and services provided should be acknowledged and they should be included in service development. Alternative ways of treatment and care should be sought locally.

(d) Patchy intervention at primary care level. A robust programme to develop primary care and mental health services is needed to shift the emphasis from secondary care to primary care.

(e) Lack of research in other areas besides schizophrenia and lack of research for smaller ethnic minority communities such as the Vietnamese, refugees and asylum seekers.

(f) Patchy development of complementary therapies. The emphasis should be on developing the range and choice of complementary therapies. There should be an awareness programme to alert the community to the choices available.

(g) Lack of understanding of the diversity within the Black and minority ethnic groups and their interpretation and presentation of mental health (as shown in Chapter 22). Ethnic minority groups are heterogenous and their diversity, lifestyles and concepts of health and disease need to be understood and included when planning service delivery.

(h) Development of the voluntary sector and consumer voices in the mental health area. It is important that the voluntary sector is developed so that it can play a full role in developing services and bring in the views of the communities to the authorities concerned.

(i) Differing views between professions, community and health service management on the way forward. It is important that all the stakeholders work together as equal partners to find solutions for mental health services locally.

(j) Need for coherent local strategies to address mental health issues.

Black and minority ethnic groups often feel that services are not for them because they are not White. They may be excluded because of direct or indirect discrimination. An example of direct discrimination might be the behaviour of staff and an example of indirect discrimination might be where services are inaccessible because they are not provided in the right language.

There are a number of key problems for the NHS and social services. There is the need to keep the issue of ethnicity to the forefront of both the development of commissioning strategies and the provision of culturally sensitive services. Although a lot of work has been done by the Department of Health to raise the profile of this issue, the unique perspective of ethnic minority people can easily be overlooked under the pressures of running of day to day services. It is also important to engage with users and carers of ethnic minority people who are likely to have strong views about what services are provided and the manner of their delivery as well as how mental health professionals may use pre-conceived ideas about people who are not from the White majority.

The following areas outline the key issues that need to be addressed in the provision of mental health care for Black and minority ethnic groups:

(a) primary care
(b) secondary care
(c) community awareness
(d) training of professionals
(e) needs assessment and commissioning
(f) research.

Primary care

As the focus for treating mental illness among ethnic minority groups has been in the secondary care area, important opportunities to diagnose mental illness early are missed in primary care settings. It is well documented that both the Asian and Caribbean populations do not consult GPs for mental disorders. In the case of Asian people, this may be due to the nature of the GP–patient interaction and poor communication (Gillam *et al*, 1989). The *Morbidity Statistics from General Practice: Fourth National Study* confirms that there was a general tendency for fewer Black people to consult for mental disorders except in the elderly, where Black men were more likely than average to consult (Office of Population Censuses and Surveys, 1995). Pathways into care are discussed in Chapters 3 and 4. Jacob *et al* (1998) reported that among 100 consecutive Asian female attendees at a GP surgery in west London, common mental disorders were documented in 37% of the patients according to research criteria, but the GP's diagnosis had a sensitivity of only 17% with a specificity of 91%. Those with common mental disorders had a significantly higher frequency of consultation.

It is important that primary care teams take a lead role in diagnosing and treating mental illness among ethnic minority groups. Following the publication of the recent NHS White Papers it is likely that this will happen. Primary care teams, particularly in inner cities, need to have appropriate training and develop a more proactive role in this area. The inner-city practices rarely have sufficient ethnic minority staff such as link-workers or nurses who can communicate with the patients effectively and understand their cultural and linguistic needs (Baxter *et al*, 1996).

To assess the health needs of the ethnic minority groups, it is important to have proper procedures and systems in place for community consultation and participation. There needs to be a clear understanding of the needs of different groups and consultation with them should be conducted on an ongoing basis. Community groups need to feel that they are partners in the process (Smaje, 1995). It is also important to recognise that when dealing with mental illness, not all groups can be representative of the views of people with mental illness, as their experience may not extend to understanding concepts of mental illness. The commissioners and providers should consult appropriate groups for this purpose. Consultation with communities is important for the primary care teams as it facilitates the efficient use of resources (see Chapters 15 and 19).

There is also a need to explain the roles of different health professionals in the primary care teams to the communities. Services such as psychotherapies, other psychological therapies, counselling and information on rights and choices in psychiatric services need to encourage people to make contact with the primary care team so that they can diagnose mental distress at an earlier stage and plan appropriate treatment.

The members of primary care teams need to create an atmosphere of understanding and build confidence within their users from ethnic minorities. They should demonstrate to minority groups that mental health and alleviation of the distress it can cause are important issues to the team. This can be shown, for example, by making available a community psychiatric nurse who speaks the service user's language and offers appropriate counselling services, or by the use of clinical psychologists offering appropriate models of intervention in stress anxiety management (Mahtani & Marks, 1994).

Improving access to health services for ethnic groups has been debated both in the community and the NHS for a very long time (Bahl, 1987). It has been highlighted that communication barriers between health professionals and the community means that appropriate information on both sides is lacking. Improved communication is a key issue which is set out in *The New NHS Charter* (Dyke, 1998) and gives a new focus to address communications with Black and minority ethnic groups.

The Department of Health has been active in the development of projects to improve communication between health professionals and service users. One example is the introduction of the link-worker scheme which is being used nationwide in different areas, the aim being to improve communication between patients and health professionals and to access appropriate health care. This should be a model for mental health services (Bahl, 1987). The Department has also commissioned a survey to identify the number of link workers in primary and secondary care and their training needs. This will help in the formulation of guidelines for the purchasers and providers.

To develop better information on mental health and services the Department of Health has funded a number of projects which are examples of good practice. These include: a video produced by Maudsley Hospital on psychiatric services in five Asian languages and Chinese, Greek, Turkish and Somali; leaflets in Asian languages on understanding the Mental Health Act; and a project to improve uptake of clinical psychology within mental health settings (further details available from the author upon request).

The White Paper *The New NHS: Modern, Dependable* (Secretary of State, 1997) highlights the development of primary care groups which will look at a range of commissioning models. Mental health care delivery must form a part of this agenda, especially in relation to vulnerable groups. The health authorities' 'health improvement programmes' should show a very focused approach to involve the voices of Black and other ethnic minority groups. They should ensure that these groups are actively involved in development and promotion of mental health care locally. The 'health action zones' should explore different models of mental health in relation to minority ethnic groups.

Secondary care

Concern has been expressed about the over-concentration of admissions for treatment at the secondary care level for some ethnic groups (Harrison *et al*, 1988). A number of explanations have been given as to the causes and reasons for apparent over-diagnosis, such as the ethnocentrism of Western psychiatry and its related professions and lack of understanding by the psychiatrists of the presenting symptoms within the cultural and religious context of the person concerned (Fernando, 1991). One of the contributing factors has been the lack of ethnic monitoring, which has prevented a better understanding of the service utilisation and attendance rates, both of which would help purchasers and providers to address this issue adequately.

The Department of Health introduced ethnicity into the Contract Minimum Data Set (CMDS) for in-patients and day cases from April 1995. The CMDS is the set of data items defined as a national standard by which providers account to commissioners for the services they have delivered under contracts. This is a major exercise which has been developed through pilot work with health authorities, professionals and through community and public consultations. The collection of ethnic group data will enable commissioners and providers to examine the uptake of services, monitor standards, identify gaps in service provision and ascertain particular needs in the secondary care area. The ethnic group classification will be consistent with national population statistics recently produced by the Office of Population Censuses and Surveys (1995).

Secondary care has not met the needs of the patients once admitted to psychiatric institutions in a culturally and ethnically sensitive manner. The secondary care provided does not take into account the wider implications of alternative medicines and therapies (MIND, 1993). In the past, hospitals have often not made efforts to talk to carers of people with mental illness, to meet communities at large to explain the secondary care services and therapy services, or to enquire from these people how services can be improved.

To improve the services provided, psychiatric teams should have a better understanding of the role of culture, race, ethnicity and the changing lifestyle of ethnic groups. Greater contact with the communities will help this process. The teams need actively to make contacts with the communities. GPs are key sources for this purpose, and secondary care providers must work closely in the community, providing services for the communities in settings where service users and their carers are comfortable, for example, primary care practices, religious places and community centres. New approaches need to be developed to offer services which demonstrate to the communities that the services are adapting to their changing needs and demands. The Department of Health funded a study, undertaken by the Bradford Community Health Trust, to look at the effectiveness of early home-based assessment of patients referred by transcultural psychiatric teams and then compare this process with the current standard assessment practice of the team (see Chapter 21).

Until recently most of the psychiatric literature concentrated upon the illness and disease model within ethnic communities. It is important that underlying social, cultural and racial factors should be studied in order to have better explanations of mental illness within psychiatry. When social factors are taken into account the effect of ethnicity *per se* may be weaker as a causative factor (Bhugra *et al*, 1997).

Communities, on the other hand, are not fully informed about the elevated admission rates to secondary care or the treatments offered, for example, in terms of the effects of medication. In the past, communities and carers have been inadequately prepared to challenge the professionals about care and treatment offered to their families. The *Cry for Change* report (Webb-Johnson, 1991, 1993; Nadirshaw, 1992) highlights the lack of trust and the suspiciousness that can develop on the part of the communities if they are not adequately equipped with information on mental illness and services provided.

Community awareness

Ethnic communities vary in their awareness of psychiatric practice in Britain. Mental illness is still a taboo word in some communities such as the Chinese (MIND, 1993). The causes of mental illness among ethnic minority groups are well documented (see Chapter 6). However, more needs to be written about individual communities' perceptions of mental illness. Some ethnic groups see psychiatric institutions as places where they will be hospitalised and will have little or no say in their treatment. Some do not see that mental illness is an area that requires professional help. They feel that it should be dealt with within the family. There has not yet been a concerted effort to promote mental health messages and awareness to ethnic communities.

The promotion of mental health awareness within the ethnic media has not been utilised as a valuable resource to communicate the importance of the subject matter. The ethnic press, like its mainstream counterparts, mainly writes negative stories about hospitals misdiagnosing mental illness. This has a detrimental effect upon community awareness, particularly when mental health is not on their agenda.

However, satellite television and Asian and African–Caribbean radio programmes provide useful and easily accessible forums in which discussion of mental health issues can be aired in the first instance. They also facilitate a wider debate within the communities.

Voluntary groups are not adequately prepared (with very few exceptions; see Chapter 20) to deal with this area of work. Some voluntary organisations do not understand how psychiatric services are provided in this country, the legislation on compulsory admissions and other important issues. This hinders them from making useful contributions towards improving services. Absence of appropriate and relevant services has led the voluntary sector to take on the role of providing mainstream services, and yet they are not equipped to do so. They have to learn by *ad hoc* experience and often work under financial constraints and heavy demands. Members of the voluntary sector should be seen as important stakeholders in planning and improving the health of Black and other minority ethnic groups – this partnership should be visible and ongoing.

The Department of Health has allocated five million pounds in the past few years to develop health work in the voluntary sector and funds have been allocated to develop mental health work: for example, funding the Confederation of Indian Organisations to identify the reasons for low uptake of psychiatric services among the Asian community and funding of the King's Fund Centre to develop a network of African and Caribbean organisations to promote effective community mental health information.

Training professionals

The need to provide better training and awareness on ethnic minority issues has been highlighted in a number of documents. Improved models of training which incorporate the health belief systems and the lifestyles of ethnic minorities and an understanding of different generations of ethnic minorities need to be developed. The training curricula should give this subject priority and should move away from an ethnocentric model (Nadirshaw, 1992). All professionals working in mental health should be trained to meet the needs of ethnic minority service users.

The development and popularity of short courses on race and cultural awareness in recent years have created the danger of marginalising the issues. Race and mental health discourse must take their place in mainstream education and must be a significant part of any professional training programme in the mental health field.

Needs assessment and commissioning

Needs assessment in psychiatric care requires involvement of all the relevant stakeholders (Rawaf & Bahl, 1998). It is important to involve commissioners, providers, the local authorities and the voluntary sector in order to develop the existing services (see Chapter 17). The commissioners and providers need to appreciate that there will be different models of delivering psychiatric care within each area.

In some areas, the voluntary sector will be strong and can make active contributions to the delivery of psychiatric care. Other areas may have developed primary or secondary care services, depending on the model chosen. It is important that all the stakeholders should be seen as active partners and their contributions should be recognised.

Since mental health is an area where ethnic groups have in the past expressed discontent with the services provided, it is important for commissioners and providers to show that the communities are involved in the needs assessment process and that all relevant groups are consulted. To develop a satisfactory needs assessment it is important to provide information on what is available within the existing psychiatric services and to equip the ethnic groups to engage in this process satisfactorily. The voluntary sector needs to be familiar with and knowledgeable about the difficulties and possibilities in delivering psychiatric care to the communities so that they can make informed decisions. Effective consultation involves:

(a) Providing full information in an accessible form.
(b) Using a wide range of techniques to facilitate participation, for example, surveys, focus groups, in-depth interviews and dialogue with user-only groups.
(c) Listening to the views of local people and involving them in continuing discussion and the decision-making processes.
(d) Acting upon views expressed.
(e) Effecting efficient feedback to those who were consulted, explaining how decisions were reached (Department of Health, 1992).

Commissioning psychiatric services is the key mechanism for changing existing psychiatric services. It is essential that the health authorities make their commissioning intentions available to the public. In drawing up commissioning intentions it is important to introduce a quality standard, based on discussions with the local groups. Commissioners should be aware of the views of the users of the services so as to improve on quality standards. An example of this is the Department of Health's funding of the Wiltshire and Bath Health Commission to purchase appropriate mental health services based upon their consultations with the community. Another example is a project funded by the Department of Health through the West Hertfordshire Community Health Trust, looking at providing recommendations to the commissioners on purchasing clinical psychology services relevant to the needs of ethnic minorities.

Research

Research in this field has also been led by health care professionals concerned about over-diagnosis of schizophrenia (Harrison *et al*, 1988). Very little research has taken place to understand the communities' perception of other types of mental illness and perceptions relating to improving early diagnosis at the primary care level. Until recently the communities' concerns about racism and discrimination within psychiatry were not addressed. However, recent studies now acknowledge this issue (Department of Health, 1992).

The lack of data on different ethnic populations has not helped researchers in the formulation of new strategies for mental health. The 1991 census provides a better indication of different ethnic populations and other social factors.

The Department of Health has been aware of service needs as well as the need to identify the prevalence of common mental disorders in minority ethnic groups. To this end, two key projects funded recently have been a study of deliberate self-harm and cultural factors in Asian women, under the aegis of the Institute of Psychiatry with other grant-giving bodies, and the commissioning of a survey by the Policy Studies Institute (Bhugra *et al*, 1996; Nazroo, 1997; also see Chapter 23). Both of the projects provide a key source of information for different types of assessment and management of common mental disorders.

Developing local mental health strategies

As the NHS White Paper (Secretary of State, 1997) provides a major focus to develop primary care, the local mental health strategy should flow out of the primary care programme and should be linked to the health improvement programmes. The health improvement programmes should ensure that multi-agency working exists at local level to provide seamless services between health, social services and other agencies. The health improvement programmes should have two major components in relation to mental health. First, the prevention of mental illness in the community, and second, the management of mental illness.

Primary care professionals should be sensitive to the lifestyles and diversity within the ethnic groups. It should be the local stakeholders, including the local Black and other minority voluntary sector, who identify imaginative ways to promote mental health in the communities.

Local communities have, for a long time, expressed discontent with mental health services both in primary and secondary care. It is important that health improvement programmes take on board the communities' views on how to improve services. The services should be audited and outcomes and successes should be disseminated to the communities. The outcomes should be evidence-based.

References

ACHESON, D. (1998) *Independent Inquiry into Inequalities in Health Report*. London: HMSO.
BAHL, V. (1987) *Asian Mother and Baby Campaign*. London: Department of Health.
BALARAJAN, R. & RALEIGH, S. V. (1993) *Health of the Nation. Ethnicity and Health – A Guide for the NHS*. London: Department of Health.
BAXTER, C., BAYLOU, A., FULLER, J., et al (1996) *The Case for the Provision of Bilingual Services Within the NHS*. London: Department of Health.
BHUGRA, D., DESAI, M. & BALDWIN, D. (1996) *Attempted Suicide in London*. London: Department of Health.
BHUGRA, D., LEFF, J., MALLET, R., et al (1997) Incidence and outcome of schizophrenia in Whites, African–Caribbeans and Asians in London. *Psychological Medicine*, **27**, 791–798.
DEPARTMENT OF HEALTH (1992) *Health of the Nation*. London: HMSO.
—— (1994) *Health of the Nation. Key Area Handbook – Mental Illness* (2nd edn). London: HMSO.
—— (1997) *Mental Health Services. The Patient's Charter*. Leeds: Department of Health.
—— (1998) *Modernising Mental Health Services: Safe, Sound and Supportive*. London: Department of Health.
DYKE, G. (1998) *The New NHS Charter: A Different Approach. Report on the New NHS Charter*. London: Department of Health.
FERNANDO, S. (ed.) (1991) *Mental Health, Race and Culture*. London: Macmillan.
GILLAM, S. J., JARMAN, B., WHITE, P., et al (1989) Ethnic differences in consultation rates in urban general practice. *British Medical Journal*, **299**, 953–957.
HARRISON, G., OWENS, D., HOLTON, A., et al (1988) A prospective study of severe mental disorders in Afro-Caribbean patients. *Psychological Medicine*, **18**, 643–657.
JACOB, K. S., BHUGRA, D., LLOYD, K., et al (1998) Common mental disorders, explanatory models and consultation behaviour among Indian women living in the UK. *Journal of the Royal Society of Medicine*, **91**, 66–71.
MAHTANI, A. & MARKS, L. (1994) Developing a primary care psychology service that is racially and culturally appropriate. *Clinical Psychology Forum*, **65**, 27–31.
MIND (1993) *Policy on Black and Minority Ethnic People and Mental Health*. MIND File Policy No. 1. London: MIND.
NADIRSHAW, Z. (1992) Therapeutic practice in multi-racial Britain. *Counselling Psychology Quarterly*, **5**, 257–261.
NATIONAL INSTITUTE FOR ETHNIC STUDIES IN HEALTH AND SOCIAL POLICY (1997) *England and Wales – The Ethnic Minority Dimension: Results from the 1991 Census*. Southall: National Institute for Ethnic Studies in Health and Social Policy.
NAZROO, J. (1997) *Ethnicity and Mental Health*. London: Policy Studies Institute.
OFFICE OF POPULATION CENSUSES AND SURVEYS (1995) *Morbidity Statistics from General Practice: Fourth National Study, 1991–1992. A study carried out by the Royal College of General Practitioners, the Office of Population Censuses and Surveys and the Department of Health*. London: HMSO.
RAWAF, S. & BAHL, V. (eds) (1998) *Assessing Health Needs of People from Minority Ethnic Groups*. London: Royal College of Physicians & Faculty of Public Health Medicine.

SECRETARY OF STATE (1997) *The New NHS: Modern and Dependable.* London: HMSO.

—— (1998*a*) *Modernising Social Services: Promoting Independence, Improving Protection, Raising Standards.* London: HMSO.

—— (1998*b*) *Our Healthier Nation.* London: HMSO.

SMAJE, C. (1995) *Health, "Race" and Ethnicity – Making Sense of the Evidence.* London: King's Fund Institute.

WEBB-JOHNSON , A. (1991) *A Cry for Change – An Asian Perspective on Developing Quality Mental Health Care.* London: Confederation of Indian Organisations.

—— (1993) *Building on Strengths – Enquiry into Health Activity in the Asian Voluntary Sector.* London: Confederation of Indian Organisations.

3   Cultural aspects of mental disorder in primary care

DAVID GOLDBERG

The referral pathways taken by patients receiving services from a mental health professional are useful in establishing the utilisation of services as well as inception rates of various diagnostic groups (Gater & Goldberg, 1991). There is a body of literature from the UK suggesting that mentally ill individuals from ethnic minorities, especially African–Caribbeans, are more likely than White people to be admitted to hospital compulsorily (Harrison *et al*, 1988; Dunn & Fahy, 1990). However, some recent studies have disputed this (King *et al*, 1994; Bhugra *et al*, 1997; also see Chapter 4). Several possible hypotheses were put forward to explain the increased rates, such as the possibility that these individuals do not use primary care facilities in the same way as the White population does.

World Health Organization (WHO) data (Ustun & Sartorius, 1995) can be used to compare English primary care attenders in south Manchester with Nigerians attending primary care clinics in Ibadan, and Indians attending similar clinics in Bangalore. However, it should not be assumed that primary care attenders in the UK of African or Asian descent will behave like those included in the WHO survey.

These pathways are likely to be influenced by conventions governing referral procedures, the relationship between primary and secondary care and simply the accessibility of services. The delay in each stage may be related to a number of factors including family support and type of symptoms.

Pathways to mental health care

There is a lot of reliable information available for Manchester, where the predominantly White population usually enters mental health care services via primary care physicians. Sixty-three per cent come via this route, with another 33% coming from hospital clinics or accident and emergency departments (Gater & Goldberg, 1991). In Bangalore and Rawalpindi the situation is different, with a substantial minority (11–17%) coming via native or religious healers, and up to 39% going directly from the community to the psychiatrist. The first port of call for a person who eventually reaches a psychiatrist in Ujung Pandang (Indonesia) is to a native or religious healer (54%); only 18% go to the local medical officer first of all and 10% are referred from hospital doctors. The equivalent figures for Manchester are 68% (visiting a GP first) and 20% (going directly to a hospital)! Virtually no-one in Manchester, Bangalore, Rawalpindi or Ujung Pandang comes into care via the police. In Nairobi, 16% of admissions are through the police or the legal system. We do not have comparable data for Ibadan or centres in the West Indies.

WHO Study

The WHO Study of Psychological Disorders in General Health Care (Ustun & Sartorius, 1995) was carried out in 15 centres across the world, and used identical methodology and procedures in each centre. Over 26 000 attenders in primary care were screened with the General Health Questionaire (GHQ–12; Goldberg & Williams, 1988), and a stratified random sample was selected in each centre for second-stage interview. Just under 5500 people were interviewed using the primary care version of the Composite International Diagnostic Interview (CIDI; Robins, 1985); these patients also completed a disability scale and were rated by the primary care physicians.

   This study provided an opportunity to investigate the pathways to care of those people who are found in primary care settings to be disturbed, rather than the small subset who were referred to the mental health services of their country. In Manchester, 95% of such people go directly to their GPs, but the situation was far more complex in Bangalore, where 20% of people were first seen by other doctors, and around 20% went from one primary care physician to another – a phenomenon known as 'doctor shopping'. It seems likely that this behaviour is determined more by the structure of the medical system than by an individual's ethnic background, but so far we have no direct evidence of this for the Asian or African–Caribbean population of the UK. There is evidence (Gater, personal communication) that in centres where primary care doctors are better able to detect mental disorders fewer people with mental illness seek care from alternative healers or seek care from a succession of different physicians (it may be that in places where mental disorder is common, primary care doctors get better at detecting it, but this is a rather simplistic explanation).

Presenting complaints and prevalence of mental disorders in primary care

About 24% of primary care attenders worldwide suffer from mental disorders recognised by the ICD–10 (World Health Organization, 1992), however, large variations were found between the centres. Few patients with mental disorders present to their doctor with psychological symptoms, except in Europe and North America. In Manchester 27% presented with psychological symptoms, but in both Ibadan and Bangalore only 4% did so. There is, therefore, some truth in the idea that Europeans are more likely to present with overtly psychological symptoms than Nigerians or Indians are – but we see that only about one in four actually do so (see Table 1). In Ibadan 21% of patients with mental disorders presented with a mixture of psychological and physical complaints, and this pattern was seen in 13.5% of those in Bangalore. However, in all the centres studied the most common presentation of these illnesses was because of pain and other physical symptoms. These accounted for 54% of the presentations in both Manchester and Bangalore, and for 68% of the presentations in Ibadan.

Prevalence across ethnic groups

The highest prevalences were seen in South America. However, of the three centres selected (see Table 2) Manchester had the highest with 26.2% of consecutive attenders suffering from confirmed mental

TABLE 1
Presenting complaints of those with ICD–10 mental disorders

	Manchester	Ibadan	Bangalore
Psychological (%)	27.0	4.8	4.0
Mixed complaints (%)	5.3	21.8	13.5
Pain (%)	21.0	36.5	39.2
Physical (%)	32.8	31.7	14.3
Other (%)	13.7	4.8	30.3

TABLE 2
Prevalence of mental disorders by gender among consecutive attenders (also showing gender ratios in three centres)

	Manchester	Ibadan	Bangalore
Males	23.7	19.0	18.1
Females	27.5	7.2	29.6
Total	26.2	10.4	23.9
Gender ratio	1.16	0.37	1.63

disorders, while the comparable figures for Bangalore and Ibadan are 23.9% and 10.4%, respectively.

A word of caution about the low Nigerian rate (see Table 2) is necessary. Medical care must be paid for at the Ibadan centre, but not in Manchester or Bangalore. It is of interest that while the male rates in the three centres are very similar (within 4% of one another), the female rates differ by more than 14%. The very low female rate in Ibadan suggests either that females are psychologically very healthy or that, if care must be paid for, the chief wage earner gets priority. Another possibility is that psychologically disordered females in this culture go to other healers.

Depression is a relatively common disorder in all these centres, although it is very common in Manchester (17%), less so in Bangalore (9%) and least common in Ibadan (4.2%). Dysthymia is very much more common (nearly 10%) in Bangalore than in either of the other centres. Despite the view that neurasthenia is a disorder more often seen in developing countries, the syndrome is in fact most common in Manchester: indeed, it is much more common in Manchester than in Shanghai. Panic disorder is also much more prevalent in Manchester than the other centres (see Table 3).

TABLE 3
Prevalence of ICD–10 mental disorders among consecutive attenders at the three centres

	Manchester	Ibadan	Bangalore
Alcohol dependence	2.2	0.4	1.4
Depression	16.9	4.2	9.1
Dysthymia	2.0	1.3	9.8
Agoraphobia	3.8	0.1	0.1
Panic disorder	3.5	0.7	1.0
Generalised anxiety disorder	7.1	2.9	8.5
'Somatic'	0.9	2.3	2.9
Neurasthenia	9.7	1.1	2.7
At least one diagnosis	26.2	10.4	23.9

Detection of disorders by doctors

Doctors in Manchester were among the best at detecting all types of mental disorders, with an overall detection rate of 63%, compared with 55% in Ibadan and only 40% in Bangalore. The reason for the lower rates is that depression is not well recognised in Ibadan, although it is easily the most common disorder; neither generalised anxiety (only 34.6%, yet 8.5% of attenders suffer from it) nor dysthymia (only 47%, yet nearly 10% of attenders suffer from it) are well recognised in Bangalore (see Table 4).

Comment

There is evidence that psychological disorders are presented to primary care physicians very differently in Manchester, Ibadan and Bangalore (Table 1). It is not known whether Nigerians or Indians living in England present differently from those in the cultures from which they originally came – this awaits further research. A comparison between Punjabi and native English presentations of mental distress in south London shows few differences, although depressive ideas, poor concentration and physical health and physical health worries were more common among the Punjabi group; the Punjabi group complained of pain symptoms more often than the English group (Bhui, personal communication). Differences between countries may reflect differences in the medical services in each place, but may also reflect the true cultural differences in the expression of psychological distress. The rarity of psychological presentations in these cultures may also reflect popular perceptions of the role of the doctor in each country studied, as well as the availability of direct referrals to the mental health services in some

TABLE 4
Percentage of mental disorders by GPs

	Manchester	Ibadan	Bangalore
Alcohol dependence	66.1	31.5	77.9
Depression	69.6	39.7	45.7
Dysthymia	80.9	90.2	46.6
Agoraphobia	70.6	38.7	46.1
Panic	72.3	67.3	34.6
Generalised anxiety disorder	72.3	67.3	34.6
One or more disorders	62.9	55.1	40.4
Two or more disorders	67.4	67.6	50.1

places. If all attenders are taken together, then psychological complaints were approximately 10% in the two South American centres, as well as in Manchester, Paris and Groningen. In centres like Seattle, Athens, Ibadan, Bangalore and Nagasaki, the psychological complaints were seen in between 1 and 2% of all attenders (see Chapter 4).

There is little doubt that the vast majority of patients follow the pathway into care described in Goldberg & Huxley's (1992) model, that is, by consulting their GPs (see Chapter 4). Inclusion of mental health care into general health care is possible by training GPs and health care staff to identify psychological symptoms (Harding *et al*, 1980; Sartorius & Harding, 1983).

By understanding pathways into care for psychiatric patients, staff training can be made more relevant, better organised and culturally sensitive – so that help can be provided sooner rather than later.

References

BHUGRA, D., LEFF, J., MALLET, R., *et al* (1997) Incidence and outcome of schizophrenia in Whites, African–Caribbeans and Asians in London. *Psychological Medicine*, **27**, 791–798.

DUNN, J. & FAHY, T. (1990) Police admissions to a psychiatric hospital. Demographic and clinical differences between ethnic groups. *British Journal of Psychiatry*, **156**, 373–378.

GATER, R. & GOLDBERG, D. (1991) Pathways to psychiatric care in south Manchester. *British Journal of Psychiatry*, **159**, 90–97.

GOLDBERG, D. & HUXLEY, P. J. (1992) *Common Mental Disorders – a Biosocial Model*. London: Routledge.

—— & WILLIAMS, P. (1988) *A Users Guide to the GHQ*. London: NFER Nelson.

HARDING, T., DE ARANGO, M., BALTAZAR, J., *et al* (1980) Mental disorders in primary health care. *Psychological Medicine*, **10**, 231–241.

HARRISON, H., OWENS, D., HOLTON, R., *et al* (1988) A prospective study of severe mental disorder in Afro-Caribbean patients. *Psychological Medicine*, **18**, 643–657.

KING, M. B., COKER, E., LEAVEY, G., *et al* (1994) Incidence of psychotic illness in London: comparison of ethnic groups. *British Medical Journal*, **309**, 1115–1119.

ROBINS, L. N. (1985) *The Composite International Diagnostic Interview, 1–2*. St Louis, MO: DIS Training Faculty and Staff, Washington University School of Medicine.

SARTORIUS, N. & HARDING, T. (1983) WHO collaborative study in strategies for extending mental health care. *American Journal of Psychiatry*, **140**, 1470–1473.

USTUN, T. & SARTORIUS, N. (1995) *Mental Health in General Health Care*. Chichester: Wiley.

WORLD HEALTH ORGANIZATION (1992) *The Tenth Revision of the International Classification of Diseases and Related Health Problems* (ICD-10). Geneva: WHO.

4 Pathways into care: an explanation of the factors that may affect minority ethnic groups

DINESH BHUGRA, RACHAEL LIPPETT and ELEANOR COLE

Kleinman (1980) defines a health care system as a mixture of health care activities dictated by the social, political and economic contexts of a culture or society. Medicine, therefore, is a cultural system – a system of symbolic meanings which are anchored in the particular arrangements of social institutions and patterns of interpersonal interactions. Illnesses, responses of individuals, their carers and society at large and the social institutions relating to them are interconnected. Health care systems include patterns of beliefs about the causes of illness, norms governing choice and evaluation of treatment, socially legitimised statuses, roles, power relationships and institutions.

At this point, it is worth drawing attention to the distinction between disease and illness which determines the levels of health-care-seeking. In anthropological terms disease is literally 'dis-ease', which refers to a malfunctioning of biological and/or psychological processes, whereas illness refers to the psychosocial experience and meaning of perceived disease (Kleinman, 1980). Illness, therefore, includes secondary personal and social responses to a primary malfunctioning in the individual's physiological or psychological status (or both) and involves processes of attention, perception, affective responses, cognitions and valuations, directed at the disease and its manifestations. Within this system are communication, and interpersonal interactions, particularly within the context of the family and social network. As Kleinman (1980) goes on to emphasise, illness is the shaping of disease into behaviour and experience created by social, personal and cultural reactions to disease. This distinction is absolutely crucial when trying to understand the pathways taken when seeking help. The development of disease into illness (at the level of the individual), and the provision of acceptable services (at health care system level) are linked in determining the pathway that a patient may follow while looking for help. Such help-seeking can be pluralistic in ethnic minorities (as indeed it can be in White communities). However, it is our contention that within a pluralistic system there is likely to be a kind of hierarchical value allocated to various kinds of help. As disease and illness are seen to be expressing different interpretations of the same clinical reality, the pathway itself is one interpretation and since we are writing from a Western perspective we shall focus on pathways into Western care systems.

Role of primary care

As highlighted in Chapter 3, investigations into the use of mental health services by ethnic minority patients indicate that primary health services are currently severely under-utilised by members of these groups. One hypothesis for this could be that the occurrence of distress is lower within the African–Caribbean community and as such Black people have far less need for the services of a general practioner (GP), hence their under-representation. Unfortunately, no more than a cursory glance through the literature demonstrates that this cannot possibly be the case. To illustrate, virtually all studies conducted have found a higher rate of psychosis among African–Caribbean people than White people. We found, for example, that rates of schizophrenia vary between 2.4 times the White rate to 18 times higher in a selected age group. A near consensus exists that levels of severe mental illness are not in fact lower but higher within the African–Caribbean community, and statistics clearly show that this has led to their over-representation in secondary care (McGovern & Cope, 1987). Thus, lower levels of distress can quickly be refuted as an interpretation of the under-utilisation of primary health care services. Nazroo (1997) reported that the prevalence of neurotic disorders such as anxiety and depression was lower in some ethnic groups than others. As these are community samples it is suggestive of differential pathways into care.

We suggest that need for mental health care is at least equally high throughout the Black community; these individuals simply follow different pathways to obtain care.

Investigation of the routes or pathways taken by people seeking help began in earnest with the publication of *Mental Illness in the Community* (Goldberg & Huxley, 1980). In it, Goldberg & Huxley proposed a five-stage model of the route from first experiencing symptoms to arrival at secondary care, and argued that each stage could be thought of as a selectively permeable filter, with some individuals having greater ability to pass through the filters than others. Although we have limited information about the model's applicability to ethnic minorities, we can argue that some of the filters will be the same even though access to the filters themselves may vary (see Fig. 1).

The first level represents the total level of morbidity in the community. Goldberg & Huxley point out that slight changes in mood, sleeping pattern and so on are common to all of us, and when an individual is able to attribute his or her 'symptoms' to an event of some kind, for example, feeling anxious before an exam, then little more attention is likely to be paid to those symptoms. Thus community surveys may pick symptoms (see Chapter 23) but not necessarily syndromes. Thus, community surveys may pick symptoms (see Chapter 23) but not necessarily syndromes. It is the inability of the individual to attribute meaning to the symptoms which renders him or her likely to move a little further along the pathway, generally by discussing the symptoms with significant others and obtaining provisional validation of the 'sick role'. If validation is given, the patient can then move on to the second stage of the model, which refers to "the total level of psychiatric morbidity among attendees in primary care settings". If the doctor should agree with the patient that he or she is not well, then professional validation is given to the symptoms: a sick note may be given out, a prescription issued

Level 1: The community

....1st **Filter**

Level 2: Total mental morbidity: attendees in primary care

....**Ability of GPs to detect disorder: 2nd Filter**

Level 3: Mental disorders identified by doctors: conspicuous psychiatric morbidity

...............................**Decision to refer to mental health services: 3rd Filter**

Level 4: Total morbidity: mental health services

....**Admission to psychiatric beds: 4th Filter**

Level 5: Psychiatric in-patient

Fig. 1
Route from experiencing symptoms to arrival at secondary care. Adapted from Goldberg &
Huxley (1980)

and the patient becomes established in the sick role. It is important to point out here that although the patient may be established in the sick role this does not necessarily mean that the psychiatric nature of the disorder has been detected, or that the patient has moved any closer to secondary services. As Goldberg has suggested in the previous chapter, a large proportion of psychiatric disorders are 'missed' by GPs, largely as a result of the tendency of patients to present their GPs with physical symptoms only. Progression to levels four and five (Fig. 1) is reliant upon the GP's recognition of the psychiatric nature of the disorder and their decision that it is necessary to refer the patient to specialist psychiatric services.

Goldberg & Huxley (1980) found that a high proportion of people suffering from a psychiatric disorder who consult their GP present only their somatic symptoms during the consultation. They speculate that this is at least partly because people assume that GPs will only be willing to attend to physical illness and will not consider psychological problems their domain. However, researchers investigating cultural variations in mental illness have amassed a body of research which suggests that the 'somatisation' of mental illness is particularly prevalent in non-Western societies and there are concerns that this leads to difficulties in detecting psychiatric illness and offering appropriate treatment.

Although Goldberg & Huxley clearly point out that movement along the pathway is contingent upon a number of factors at each stage, and that in every case progression to the next level is only one of a number of decisions which could be made, they also state that at least two-thirds of those who arrive at psychiatric services have taken one common pathway – they have presented to their GP and been referred on. Only a very small proportion of people reach services via alternative routes.

Mental health policy has developed since the 1980s. Mental health is now one of the first two National Service Frameworks. The Framework will cover the full spectrum of mental health services including the primary care services. Publication of these social standards is expected in 1999. In addition the NHS White Papers for England, Wales and Scotland and the Green Paper highlight the importance of prevention and primary health care in mental health service delivery.

Seeking help

Research (much less British research) into the help-seeking behaviour of minority ethnic groups is scant, but investigations conducted in the USA suggest that the majority of Black people with mental health problems either seek no help at all or utilise the traditional health care sector and informal social support networks (Neighbors, 1985). As such, we seek to establish that the 'alternative pathway hypothesis' is one of the explanations for the under-representation of Black patients in primary care and to investigate the reasons why this should be so.

Assessments and diagnoses are made by professionals across agencies who are very often influenced by assumptions and stereotyped views. This may explain why service delivery to Black and Asian people is often inappropriate. The system has failed to gain their trust which discourages many from seeking help at an early stage or, indeed, at all.

It is our contention that any adequate explanation of help-seeking behaviour needs to account for factors operating at both the individual and cultural levels, to consider factors pertinent to the social institutions themselves and to appreciate the interaction between the three (Fig. 2).

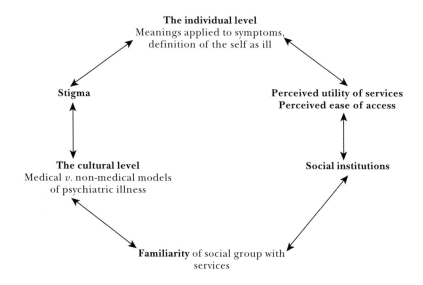

FIG. 2
Interaction between social and individual levels

The individual level

Factors operating at the individual level correspond to Goldberg & Huxley's first level: the individual in the community attempting to apply meaning to the disturbing symptoms that he or she is experiencing. For the individual to make any progression along the pathway to care the first step is for the symptoms to be interpreted as indicative of an illness. Janis & Rodin (1979) state that the amount of pain and distress a person suffers is largely dependent on the cognitions and labels that are applied to the condition, rather than purely and simply the intrinsic properties of the condition itself. In order to appreciate the way in which individuals come to view themselves as having a mental health problem it is necessary to understand the individual's cognitive processes.

For an individual to be able to acknowledge a problem, view it in mental health terms and accept professional referral, that person must have some acceptance of psychiatry, what it can offer, treatments available as well as the success rates of such treatments. Additionally, the individual must view mental health problems as illnesses, rather than a sign of weakness or a character defect. But although many people may outwardly state that a mental health problem is nothing to be ashamed of, their attitude changes when they are personally affected (Gurin *et al*, 1960).

People are generally not even aware of their resistance to seeking help, for defence mechanisms operate at quite a deep level. It is not that people recognise that they have a serious problem and refuse to seek help, but that defence mechanisms cause people to convince themselves that they do not have a problem, and therefore do not need help. This is quite likely to arise out of a fear of the stigma that mental illness can bring; individuals find it hard to reconcile their self-image with the unhappy and ineffectual individual that is their picture of a mentally ill person. In a review of the literature discussing psychiatric stigma in non-Western societies, Fabrega (1991) confirms that such societies tend to have both medical and non-medical frameworks for dealing with psychiatric illness and the non-medical frameworks can encompass supernatural, religious, moralistic or magical interpretations of the 'symptoms'. Fabrega notes that in these societies there is a wide variation in the range of possible reactions to psychiatric disorders; some are treated no differently to physical illnesses. However, if conditions become chronic and do not appear to respond to treatment, there is an increased tendency for them to be explained as a result of sorcery, witchcraft or punishment for breaking moral taboos – it is then that the individual can come to be seen as blameworthy in some way and socially stigmatised. It is currently unclear whether stigmatisation is a particular problem among ethnic minorities in Britain today. One way forward may be to uncover the processes by which individuals come to define themselves as mentally ill, and their beliefs surrounding mental illness, and how it should be dealt with. This would need to be seen in conjunction with Nazaroo's (1997) findings that rates of neurotic disorder in the minority ethnic groups are lower than in the White group.

In an investigation into the cognitive structures that mediate illness labeling and help-seeking processes, Angel & Thoits (1987) point out that that the perspective of the individual and his or her interpretations of physical and emotional states has been neglected by researchers, who have tended to favour sociological/ anthropological-style examinations of the impact of the wider culture on these factors. As such, there is substantial research evidence that individuals living in traditional cultures exhibit quite different health and illness behaviours to those in modern industrialised societies, but there is little knowledge about the extent to which traditional beliefs continue to influence individuals' cognitions when they move out of a traditional culture into contemporary Western society.

Cultures vary in the extent to which they lead individuals to be aware of bodily states. Zola (1972) found that in consultation Italians are more likely to report a number of symptoms, in contrast to the Irish, who report only a few. Tendencies towards introspection are more common among females and Jewish people. Therefore it appears that culture plays a role in the beginning, in sensitising the individual to physical and emotional states (Hansell & Mechanic, 1985). The interpretation of a sensation as a symptom and as serious or non-serious will depend to some extent on the prevalence of those types of sensations in the culture as a whole; the more widespread a symptom is within a social group, the less likely a person is to attribute significance to it. The social desirability or undesirability of the symptom will affect the likelihood of the individual seeking provisional validation of the symptoms from friends and relatives, and his or her feelings about acknowledging the problem and seeking help. From this it is clear that the negotiation of a pathway to care involves decisions made by the individual and his or her carer which are strongly affected by his or her culture.

The cultural level

The patient does not necessarily negotiate the pathway to care alone, but does so under the influence of significant others in his or her life. Indeed, Cole *et al* (1995) found that one of the most significant factors governing the pathway taken to receive care was the presence of a carer of some kind, to help negotiate help-seeking. Involvement of friends or relatives was found to be strongly associated with avoidance of compulsory admission, or coming to the attention of the police. Many studies suggest that, irrespective of ethnicity, people will turn to their natural support systems first – turning to statutory organisations only as a last resort (Gourash, 1978). Kleinman (1980) observes that although the popular sphere of health care is the largest part of any system it is the least studied and most poorly understood. Studies undertaken in the USA and Taiwan indicate that 70–90% of all illness episodes are managed within the popular sector (Zola, 1972, 1973).

It is here that cultural factors come into play, since the person's friends and relatives will express beliefs and standards that are representative of the world view of the larger social group. Some non-Western cultures encompass a variety of different beliefs about mental health and its origins, ranging from supernatural models (spirit intrusion, spirit possession, soul loss) to religious models (moral integrity, ethical conduct) and naturalistic explanations (principles of balance, yin and yang), although these models are not necessarily applicable to second- and third-generation British Black people who were born and educated in a Western society. In all of these examples problems are not conceived in mental health terms, and as such it would clearly not be logical for a mental health professional to be approached. But particularly among groups who believe that mental health is achieved through a system of balance and the thinking of harmonious thoughts, the notion of dwelling on a problem would probably seem quite threatening, and the mainstream mental health service approach directly opposes their expectations of care.

The folk sector (non-professional, non-bureaucratic, specialist) merges into both the popular and professional sectors. Folk medicine is a mixture of many different components. As Kleinman (1980) points out, in some cultures popular and folk sectors may constitute the only health care system available. Folk medicine is frequently classified into sacred and secular parts, but this itself may be blurred The efficacy of folk healing presents a serious question for the care-givers working in professional sectors. It is difficult to ascertain its efficacy and if folk healing becomes a part of the statutory service will it retain the same definition? The structural components of folk, personal and professional sectors overlap, and the models of care can be pluralistic if the patients and their carers are keen to use these.

Repeated studies have found that in developing countries a traditional healer will often be consulted first, in preference to a medical doctor. This is likely to be a direct result of mental health problems being viewed in non-medical terms, but it has been found that this is particularly the case in countries where psychiatric services are less well resourced (Gater *et al*, 1991). Interestingly, they also noted that those seeking help from native healers often travelled a recursive pathway and experienced greater delays. If we accept that in other countries alternative pathways are taken, it seems understandable that when immigrants move to the developed world they bring such a pattern of interaction with them. The role of pathways into care (as proposed by the World Health Organization) in developing services is worth remembering, especially in relation to diagnosis (Bhugra, 1997).

Research suggests that even in Western societies like the USA a far greater proportion of Black people with serious problems will approach 'informal networks' rather than the mental health sector, and in particular they are more likely to approach Black churches; Neighbors (1985) found that nearly 20% of the Black people in his study sought help from a minister.

Kadushin (1969) has suggested that the propensity to approach psychiatric services is partly governed by the familiarity of those in the individual's social network with the services themselves. If we accept that many individuals from minority ethnic cultures view their problems in non-medical terms and often have a negative perception of psychiatric services, then the likelihood of any member engaging with mental health services is slim and a vicious circle ensues. It is also reasonable that those who are familiar with services who have suffered such a negative experience are unlikely to recommend the services to their friends or wish to encounter the services again themselves.

The social institution

Social institution theories purport to explain help-seeking behaviour by examining the availability and access of health services and the quality of care that is given. How do elements of the mental health system either promote or prevent service use? It has been suggested that, in cities, proximity to transport services and a feeling of safety in the area in which the service is located combine to create a new variable, perceived access, which is more important than actual geographical location. In setting up community services for ethnic minorities the Royal College of Psychiatrists has recommended certain criteria (Bhugra *et al*, 1995). The services have to be accessible, acceptable, user-friendly and culturally sensitive. Many prospective patients may have no idea where services are geographically located and, even when they do, transport costs and travelling times are off-putting to them.

The organisational approach focuses specifically on those aspects of the service which are actually being delivered and not the 'hidden' aspects of the service. Professional staff from ethnic minorities are under-represented generally in psychiatric services. Wu & Windle (1980) suggest that, quite apart from the linguistic problems that can arise when the therapist and patient come from a different culture, there are particular difficulties involved in establishing a therapeutic relationship when each holds a different world view and philosophy of life, and the goals and processes considered appropriate by the therapist may be antithetical and useless to the patient (Ibrahim, 1985). Together, such factors may combine to affect the pathway into care that an African–Caribbean person may take.

There is controversy over the quality of the services that Black people receive once they are actually in care, and again the issue is hampered by a lack of research in Britain. However, a report issued by the Mental Health Foundation (1995) described the mental health care received by ethnic minorities as "incomplete and inconsistent" and complained of "...worrying differences between the ways in which White people and those from ethnic minorities receive care...". In a separate piece of research, Geraghty (1985) found that White patients were almost twice as likely to be offered psychotherapy and were on average seen for more sessions.

Conclusion

Any adequate model of help-seeking behaviour needs to encompass individual variables, which are in turn impinged upon by cultural factors, both of which will be affected by variables related to the nature of mental health services and their delivery.

Help-seeking behaviour is determined by personal/individual and social/cultural factors. We need to understand both factors and their interactions in determining the points of entry into professional health care systems.

References

ANGEL, R. & THOITS, P. (1987) The impact of culture on the cognitive structure of illness. *Culture, Medicine and Psychiatry*, **11**, 465–494.

BHUGRA, D. (1997) Setting up services: Cross-cultural issues. *International Journal of Social Psychiatry*, **3**, 16–28.

——, Bridges, K. & Thompson, C. (1995) *Caring for a Community*. Council Report CR36. London: Royal College of Psychiatrists.

COLE, E., LEAVEY, G., KING, M., *et al* (1995) Pathways to care for patients with a first episode of psychosis. A comparison of ethnic groups. *British Journal of Psychiatry*, **167**, 770–776.

FABREGA, H. (1991) Psychiatric stigma in non-Western societies. *Comprehensive Psychiatry*, **32**, 534–551.

GATER, R., ALMEIDA, E. & DE SOUSA, B. (1991) The pathways to psychiatric care: A cross-cultural study. *Psychological Medicine*, **21**, 761–774.

GERAGHTY, W. (1985) Ethnicity as a variable in the provision and delivery of service in an inner city psychology service. *Counseling Psychologist*, **13**, 4–16.

GOLDBERG, D. P. & HUXLEY, P. (1980) *Mental Illness in the Community*. London: Tavistock.

GOURASH, N. (1978) Helpseeking: A review of the literature. *American Journal of Community Psychology*, **6**, 413–424.

GURIN, G., VEROFF, J. & FELD, S. (1960) *Americans View Their Mental Health*. New York: Basic Books.

HANSELL, S. & MECHANIC, D. (1985) Introspectiveness and adolescent symptom-reporting. *Journal of Human Stress*, **11**, 165–176.

IBRAHIM, F. (1985) Effective cross cultural counseling and psychotherapy: A framework. *Counseling Psychologist*, **13**, 625–636.

JANIS, I. & RODIN, J. (1979) Attribution, control and decision making: Social psychology and health care. In *Health Psychology* (eds G. C. Stone, F. Cohen, & N. Adler). San Francisco, CA: Jossey-Bass.

KADUSHIN, C. (1969) *Why People Go to Psychiatrists*. New York: Atherton Press.

KLEINMAN, A. (1980) *Patients and Their Healers in the Context of Culture*. Berkeley, CA: University of California Press.

McGOVERN, D. & COPE, R. V. (1987) First admission rates for first and second generation Afro-Caribbeans. *Social Psychiatry*, **22**, 139–149.

MENTAL HEALTH FOUNDATION (1995) *Mental Health in Black and Minority Ethnic People*. London: Mental Health Foundation.

NAZROO, J. (1997) *Ethnicity and Mental Health*. London: Policy Studies Institute.

NEIGHBORS, H. W. (1985) Seeking professional help for personal problems: Black Americans' use of health and mental health services. *Community Mental Health Journal*, **21**, 156–166.

WU, I. & WINDLE, C. (1980) Ethnic specificity in the relative minority use and staffing of community mental health centres. *Community Mental Health Journal*, **16**, 156–168.

ZOLA, I. K. (1972) Medicine as an institution of social control. *Sociological Review*, **20**, 487–504.

—— (1973) Pathways to the doctor – from person to patient. *Social Science and Medicine*, **7**, 677–684.

5 Epidemiological factors in research with ethnic minorities

JULIAN LEFF

Attempting to study the epidemiological data on psychiatric conditions across cultures is problematic. Ethnicity is only one of the variables (see Chapter 1), and instruments used to measure psychopathology carry problems of category fallacy, as outlined by Kleinman (1977) and discussed elsewhere in this volume. However, we need epidemiological data to plan services and attempt to understand the aetiology of some conditions. There are several methodological problems in carrying out epidemiological studies (Leff, 1988). I aim to illustrate some of the difficulties using some British studies as examples.

Problems

Epidemiological studies can afford us some interesting insights into the possible causes of mental illness. A good example is the study conducted by the World Health Organization on the incidence of schizophrenia across a variety of cultures (Jablensky *et al*, 1992). The main publications concentrate on incidence, that is, the first contact rate, for what is sometimes called 'nuclear schizophrenia'. This is the most easily recognisable form, which has symptoms defined by Schneider (1957). The rates vary within a fairly narrow range, the lowest being in Aarhus at 7 per 100 000 and the highest in Nottingham, UK at 14 per 100 000. The difference between these rates is not statistically significant, indicating an unusual pattern for schizophrenia, since no other disease has the same incidence rate all over the world. However, if 'fringe schizophrenia' is considered, that is, not the central syndrome but other delusions and hallucinations, the variation is much bigger, from a low of 3.8 in Aarhus to 23.5 in the rural areas of Chandigarh in India, which is a highly significant variation. A variation in rates of this magnitude can provide clues to the potential causes of the illness, because it is then possible to compare the populations and determine other differences between them.

The rate of illness is quite simply a vulgar fraction – the number of cases over the size of the population. However, in calculating rates there are a great many problems to overcome. First, when considering the numerator, cases may be missed because they may not present to the service. This is a much more important issue with neuroses than psychoses, since most people with schizophrenia or a manic–depressive illness are not containable within the family, and they eventually come to the attention of health or social services. The situation with neuroses is quite different, as will be discussed below.

The non-applicability of diagnostic concepts across cultures is a difficult issue to deal with Kleinman (1977) called it 'category fallacy'. A good example is the concept of depression, which has been developed from clinical experience in Western cultures. It cannot be automatically assumed that the concept will transfer simply to another culture and that it will be possible to search for all the cases of depression in this other cultural group. This might be an issue even with psychosis, a point raised by Littlewood & Lipsedge (1981) in their classic paper in which they suggested that there was a misdiagnosis of African–Caribbean patients by White psychiatrists. Their study, based on 37 patients admitted to a hospital in London, found that a change of diagnosis was twice as common with African–Caribbean patients as it was with the native White patients, and it was as common to change the diagnosis from schizophrenia to another illness, as from another diagnosis to schizophrenia. They also noticed that a higher proportion of the African–Caribbean patients' illnesses were complicated by religious issues (40% compared with 14% of the native White patients) and they raised the question of whether psychiatrists are capable of distinguishing strong religious beliefs of a minority sect from actual mental illness. Their suggestion of misdiagnosis has become part of the popular ideation about mental illness and has become a political issue about the social control of Black people by the psychiatric system. However, a careful look at what Littlewood & Lipsedge actually found suggests a different interpretation. When they looked at 36 subjects, of whom 20 were African–Caribbean, four were West African, eight were European and eight were native White patients, all had religious issues involved in their illnesses. They found that there was a predominance of females in the sample group: 70% of the African–Caribbean and West African patients were female compared with 33% of the European and native White patients. They tried to perform a standardised assessment using the Present State Examination (PSE; Wing *et al*, 1974), and found that 12 of the African–Caribbean patients initially could not be rated. In other words, the illness was so disturbing to the patient that they could not even answer the interviewer's questions. However, of those who could be examined, all had a psychotic class of illness within the standardised system of diagnosis: none of the patients was classed as neurotic or normal. The issue really concerns the type of psychosis the person is suffering from, not whether or not the person is psychotic. The findings of Littlewood & Lipsedge (1981) have been misinterpreted by both the lay public and some professionals, who have indicated that there is confusion as to whether people have psychosis or not. In fact, misdiagnosis, when dealing with psychosis, may not be as serious a problem as has been thought previously. However, it emerges as a problem when focusing on neurosis, and this is partly to do with the various pathways to specialist care in developed and developing countries.

As discussed in Chapters 3 and 4, consideration of pathways to care for the mainstream White culture in the UK indicates that relatively few patients go through alternative medicine to get to the hospital specialist; the majority consult their general practioner (GP), who refers only 5% of these patients to a hospital specialist. As highlighted by Goldberg (Chapter 3), in a developing country, a large number of people are seen by a traditional healer and some by medical assistants, who may be working at the village level. A major problem concerns the population on which researchers have developed their assessments of symptoms. In the West, the PSE (Wing *et al*, 1974) was developed on hospital cases and has since been applied at the general population level. The General Health Questionnaire (GHQ; Goldberg, 1972) was developed around GP cases and then used at a higher level to assess people in hospital, and also at a lower level to look at the general population. Thus, there may be all kinds of odd complaints or symptoms in the general population that do not get incorporated in the standardised instruments. It becomes even more biased when these instruments are used in a developing country or with people who come from a developing country, whose complaints are well recognised by the traditional healer but bear very little relationship to what people in a Western country will complain of to their GPs. We know very little about what traditional healers do or how they diagnose illness, or the kinds of complaints that are presented to them. There have been some attempts in developing countries to produce relevant scales. Some of these have been developed in India, and one in China (Leff, 1988), but the researchers have all started at the level of the hospital specialist, and have developed their instruments on the basis of patients who have reached this level. This starting point is too specialised because patients who reach the hospital specialist have already passed through several filters which may hold back people with complaints that do not fit Western models.

Problems also arise with the denominator, in particular with the age structure of the population. It is very important to standardise for age when calculating rates of illness. An instructive example is provided by comparing the age distribution of males in the 1971 census for England and Wales with that of White and African–Caribbean residents in Camberwell, London (Leff *et al*, 1976). The age distribution shows a trough for the England and Wales population census and also for the White males in Camberwell for the middle years of life. In contrast, there is a large peak for African–Caribbean men of the same age range. This is because able-bodied African–Carribean people came to the UK in the 1950s; they were recruited by London Transport and by nursing agencies, who brought in people of working age. In 1971, there were very few elderly African–Caribbean people in the UK population and also few in the younger age groups. This distribution, of course, is gradually changing. However, looking at schizophrenia at that point in time, there was a much bigger population of African–Caribbean people likely to devlop the illness compared with White people, because the 20s to 40s age group contains the highest incidence of new cases of schizophrenia. It is important to standardise for age, and some of the influential studies carried out previously did not do so.

The final problem is unrecorded people. We have to rely on census figures to provide a base population. Despite its faults, the 1991 census allowed for self-ascribed ethnicity, and no other census has ever done so. Consequently, it is the first time that a direct measure of the size of the ethnic population has been available. However, there was a sizeable group of people who did not want to register, and it is difficult to know how to estimate the number involved. The Office of Population Censuses and Surveys (1994) has estimated that no more than 10% of the population was missed, and that there was no ethnic bias among the unregistered, but there are reasons to doubt the validity of this estimate. One of the main problems regarding unregistered people is a political one, namely that people who are illegal UK residents are unlikely to register.

Some solutions

Beiser *et al* (1972) studied the Serer people of Senegal. They interviewed chiefs, native healers and priests, and asked them to identify the categories and disorders they recognised. Then they interviewed sufferers of *O Dof*, a disorder where people became mad as a result of spirit attack. They were administered a structured Western interview and also an unstructured clinical interview, in an effort to make the assessment as broad as possible and to try to avoid the preconceptions of a Western instrument. It was found that, within the general category of *O Dof*, there was a class of disorder called *Pobouh Lang*, which was applied to people who ate earth. People who eat earth among the Serer are considered to be quite normal if they are pregnant women or young unweaned children, but if they are in any other category of the population they are considered to be suffering from a disorder. This would not have been noticed using the GHQ or the PSE, or any other Western instrument. This is an example of the way in which our own system narrows our thinking, so that we believe that we understand how to investigate mental illness across cultural boundaries. As noted earlier, this is a particular problem when we come to consider neurotic conditions. Rates of depression show enormous variations between one culture and another. For example, psychiatric illness in GP attenders detected using the GHQ was found to affect 50% of those in Santiago in Chile, 30% in Rio de Janeiro, but only 7% in Shanghai. The degree of variation in the amount of psychiatric morbidity seen in primary care attenders indicates either that neurosis is remarkably different in its frequency in these different cultures, or that the categories of neurotic illness do not apply to all cultures. It is instructive to concentrate on depression, taking into consideration the influence that culture has both on the way depression is experienced and the manner in which it is presented, whether to a traditional healer or a Western-style doctor.

There is variable emphasis on somatic versus psychological symptoms (see Chapters 3 and 4). The purely psychological presentation of depression is rare enough in the West – it is almost never seen in a developing country. This is reflected in the use of language; there are some languages which have no obvious equivalents for 'depression' and 'anxiety'. It is possible to find phrases that partly replace depression or anxiety, but complications arise when they are translated back. In the World Health Organization (1973) study of schizophrenia, the PSE, which was developed in English, was translated into seven other languages, including Yoruba, a Nigerian language. Translation of the Yoruba phrase for depression back into English resulted in the expression 'the heart is weak'. It may or may not have a direct relationship to depression, but it clearly has a very strong somatic reference. Consequently, one set of problems arises from the language into which the instrument is translated. Another very interesting issue has been raised by Obeyesekere (1985) in Sri Lanka concerning what he calls "the work of culture". He proposes that cultures have different ways of helping individuals cope with loss. For example, among the Kaluli in New Guinea, if a person loses a wife or a pig or any valued possessions, they expect to be compensated for their loss by society. The reaction is not one of grief but of anger: "Look what's happened to me, do something about it"; and the society comes together and compensates the aggrieved person in some way for their loss (Schieffelin, 1985). In Iran, grief is a communal act, which centres on the issue of martyrdom. The martyr/hero theme in Muslim culture is very strong; martyrdom is a holy state. So, if a person loses a loved one, the whole community participates in the support system (Good *et al*, 1985). Obeyesekere (1985) describes a particular kind of Buddhism in Sri Lanka, which encourages meditation on the worthlessness of life: that we are all just clay vessels with nothing inside and, when the vessels break, they are destroyed and it is of no significance. This is, of course, denying the value of loss, if we look at it in Western psychological terms. Obeyesekere considers that this is one way of coming to terms with loss, and views our attempts in the West to deal with loss as a medicalisation of distress, since we call it an illness, namely depression. One consequence is that, when Westerners study other cultures which have very different ways of dealing with loss, they may not see depression or recognise it at all because they have different coping mechanisms for dealing with loss.

Implications of epidemiology

Recently, we studied Ealing, London (Bhugra *et al*, 1997). We chose this area because it has a large Asian population, as well as a reasonably large group of African–Caribbean residents. We also included the area of south Southwark because of the large African–Caribbean population living there. The African–Caribbean rate of incidence for nuclear schizophrenia (patients with Schneider's first-rank symptoms) is about twice as high as for the White and Asian people, who have similar rates of incidence. The pattern for fringe or broad schizophrenia is different, with the Asian rate half-way between the White and the African–Caribbean rates of incidence. When nuclear and fringe schizophrenia are combined to form a broad grouping, the African–Caribbean group stands out as having a rate twice that of the other two ethnic groups, which is a significant difference (Bhugra *et al*, 1997).

The magnitude of the difference in incidence rates is a starting point in the search for the causes of schizophrenia. In the study mentioned above (Bhugra *et al*, 1997) there were far more Asian patients over the age of 30 years than there are White or African–Caribbeans, far more of them are married, and a much higher proportion of the Asian patients were not born in the UK –

88% compared with 8% of the White group. Only 29% of the African–Caribbean people were born abroad, so the Asian population appears to be very different when considering all these factors. Since the Asian rate of incidence in our study was not different from the White rate of incidence, the demographic differences are not very interesting, from the point of view of the cause of schizophrenia. What is interesting is the one factor on which the African–Caribbean people differ from both the Asian and White people – unemployment. The proportions of unemployed were: 50% of the Asian patients, 55% of the White patients and 82% of the African–Caribbean patients. This suggests that there may be a factor in the experience of being unemployed that is linked to the origins of schizophrenia.

This is not the first time that this suggestion has been made (see Bhugra, 1993 for a review; Warner, 1994). Controversy has raged for years over the relationship between unemployment, low socio-economic status and schizophrenia. Our findings suggest that this is a fruitful area in which to explore causal issues in the origins of schizophrenia (see Chapter 23).

Data from a one-year follow-up study of patients with first-onset schizophrenia (Bhugra *et al*, 1997) show that the differences in outcome are dramatic. Poor outcome was defined as relapse, suicide or failure to recover from the initial episode and was found in 24% of White, 17% of Asian and 60% of African–Caribbean patients. This finding may have nothing to do with the origins of schizophrenia, but rather with the relationship of the patients to the service: the experience they have had of their in-patient stay, their satisfaction with the treatment given, and how these have affected their compliance with after-care. Patient satisfaction is now regarded as a salient indicator of performance of the service. It was not measured in this study, but it is being assessed in our current study of the same area. The poor outcome of first-onset African–Caribbean patients is not only important theoretically, but it is of enormous practical importance. There are momentous implications for psychiatric services, both in terms of the volume of care needed and the quality of the service provided.

Conclusions

The differences between rates in psychoses and neuroses (see Chapter 7) are suggestive of many possible explanations. It is likely that there are genuine differences in rates among many ethnic groups. Furthermore, instruments of assessment may not measure what they are purporting to measure. It is also likely that the idioms of distress vary and, because of linguistic, semantic and conceptual differences, this is not identified. Another possible hypothesis is that the samples are not adequately representative. It makes sense for clinicians and researchers alike to be aware of these issues when collecting and interpreting data.

References

BEISER, M., RAVEL, J-L., COLLOMB, H., *et al* (1972) Assessing psychiatric disorder among the Serer of Senegal. *Journal of Nervous and Mental Diseases*, **154**, 141–151.

BHUGRA, D. (1993) Poverty, unemployment and homelessness. In *Principles of Social Psychiatry* (eds D. Bhugra & J. Leff). Oxford: Blackwell Scientific.

–––, LEFF, J., MALLETT, R., *et al* (1997) Incidence and outcome of schizophrenia in Whites, African–Caribbeans and Asians in London. *Psychological Medicine*, **27**, 791–798.

GOLDBERG, D. P. (1972) *The Detection of Psychiatric Illness by Questionnaire (GHQ)*. Maudsley Monograph 21. Oxford: Oxford University Press.

GOOD, B. J., GOOD, M. & MORADI, R. (1985) The interpretation of Iranian depressive illness and dysphoric affect. In *Culture and Depression: Studies in the Anthropology and Cross-Cultural Psychiatry of Affect and Disorder* (eds A. Kleinman & B. Good), pp. 369–428. Berkeley, CA: University of California Press.

JABLENSKY, A. M., SARTORIUS, N., ERNBERG, G., *et al* (1992) Schizophrenia: manifestations, incidence and course in different cultures. A World Health Organization ten-country study. *Psychological Medicine*, Monograph Supplement **20**, 1–97.

KLEINMAN, A. (1977) Depression somatisation and the new cross-cultural psychiatry. *Social Science and Medicine*, **11**, 3–10.

LEFF, J. (1988) *Psychiatry Around the Globe*. London: Gaskell.

–––, FISCHER, M. & BERTELSEN, A. (1976) A cross-national epidemiological study of mania. *British Journal of Psychiatry*, **129**, 428–442.

LITTLEWOOD, R. & LIPSEDGE, M. (1981) Some social and phenomenological characteristics of psychotic immigrants. *Psychological Medicine*, **11**, 289–302.

OBEYESEKERE, G. (1985) Depression, Buddhism and the work of culture in Sri Lanka. In *Culture and Depression* (eds A. Kleinman & B. Good), pp. 134–152. Berkeley, CA: University of California Press.

OFFICE OF POPULATION CENSUSES AND SURVEYS (1994) *1991 Census User Guide. No 58. Undercoverage in Great Britain*. Scotland: General Register Office.

SCHIEFFELIN, E. L. (1985) The cultural analysis of depressive affect: an example from New Guinea. In *Culture and Depression: Studies in the Anthropology and Cross-Cultural Psychiatry of Affect and Disorder* (eds A. Kleinman & B. Good), pp. 101–133. Berkeley, CA: University of California Press.

SCHNEIDER, K. (1957) Primare and Sekundare Symptome bei der Schizophrenie. *Fortschritte der Neurologie und Psychiatrie*, **25**, 487–490.

WARNER, R. (1994) *Recovery from Schizophrenia: Psychiatry and Political Economy* (2nd edn). London: Routledge.

WING, J. K., COOPER, J. E. & SARTORIUS, N. (1974) *Measurement and Classification of Psychiatric Symptoms: An Instruction Manual for the PSE and Catego Program*. London: Cambridge University Press.

WORLD HEALTH ORGANIZATION (1973) *The International Pilot Study of Schizophrenia*. Vol 1. Geneva: WHO.

6 Risk factors for psychosis in the UK African–Caribbean population

KWAME McKENZIE and ROBIN M. MURRAY

There have been many reports of an increased incidence of schizophrenia and mania in people of African–Caribbean origin living in the UK (Leff *et al*, 1976; Harrison *et al*, 1988; Wessely *et al*, 1991; King *et al*, 1994; Van Os *et al*, 1996*a,b*; Bhugra *et al*, 1997). Initially, rates of 6–18 times that in the White population were quoted, but more recently figures two to three times greater have been reported (Leff *et al*, 1976; Harrison *et al*, 1988; Wessely *et al*, 1991; King *et al*, 1994; Van Os *et al*, 1996*a,b*; Bhugra *et al*, 1997). The decline in the magnitude of the reported excess incidence may be due to a real fall in the incidence of psychosis in African–Caribbean people in the UK, or it may be due to improvements in the methodology of the studies. The research has many shortfalls, including sampling bias and difficulties in enumeration of the African–Caribbean population in the UK; these have been widely discussed in the literature (Sashidharan, 1993) and attempts have been made to correct for possible errors in estimations (Van Os *et al*, 1996*a,b*).

There is, of course, a fundamental problem with the very term African–Caribbean (see Chapter 1 for problems regarding definitions). However, in the research we quote, in 90% of cases either the patients or their parents were born in Jamaica.

In spite of all the above difficulties, even the most sceptical of commentators now concede that African–Caribbean individuals living in the UK have an increased risk of being diagnosed as having psychosis, even if the size of this increase may be a matter for debate (Sashidharan, 1993). Our research has aimed to elucidate possible causes for the increased incidence (McKenzie *et al*, 1995*b*; Hutchinson *et al*, 1996). Identification of specific risk factors for psychosis in the African–Caribbean population could not only lead to the development of

48

preventive strategies, but could also provide information for the wider debate on the aetiology of the psychoses (see Chapter 5).

Biological risk factors, such as genetic predisposition and neuro-developmental impairment, are generally considered of crucial importance for the development of psychosis; most present-day researchers consider that social factors are likely to play a precipitating rather than a fundamentally causal role in the development of schizophrenia in White people (Murray *et al*, 1992). Paradoxically, much of the debate about the reasons for the increased incidence of schizophrenia in the African–Caribbean population in the UK has centred on the possible risk-increasing effects of social or cultural factors such as social stress, culturally mediated substance misuse, oppression and migration (Littlewood & Lipsedge, 1981; Fernando, 1988; Eagles, 1991; Sashidharan, 1993).

Our aim is to look at the social and biological risk factors for psychosis that are thought of as being important in the White population, and investigate their relative importance in the African–Caribbean population in the UK. Are these factors more, less or equally important in the African–Caribbean population in the UK, and do they account for the increased incidence of psychoses (McKenzie *et al*, 1995*b,c*; Hutchinson *et al*, 1996)?

Misdiagnosis

The idea that misdiagnosis was inflating the incidence of schizophrenia was put forward particularly by Littlewood & Lipsedge (1981); they considered that many African–Caribbean people diagnosed as suffering from schizophrenia were really suffering from brief reactive psychoses which were misdiagnosed. However, other researchers have challenged this idea (see Chapter 5). Lewis *et al* (1990) sent case vignettes about patients to psychiatrists practising in Britain, and asked for their diagnoses. The ethnicity of the patients in the case histories was randomly changed from White to African–Caribbean while all other clinical information remained the same. The results indicated that the psychiatrists were more reluctant to make the diagnosis of schizo-phrenia in African–Caribbean than in White patients.

Other researchers investigating cross-cultural incidence rates have tried to eradicate misdiagnosis by using operational criteria to define schizophrenia (Harrison *et al*, 1988; Wessely *et al*, 1991; King *et al*, 1994; Bhugra *et al*, 1997). However, this may have inadvertently introduced bias into their studies because none of the systems used for diagnosis had been rigorously tested on a UK African–Caribbean population. There are also anthropological arguments against applying the Western concept of schizophrenia to people from other cultures (Fernando, 1988). Furthermore, the current practice of studying single diagnostic categories of questionable validity may introduce selection bias (Robins & Guze, 1970), especially as the excess risk for psychosis in the African–Caribbean population in the UK has not been shown to be disorder-specific.

In our own studies, we have endeavoured to investigate psychosis in general rather than just schizophrenia. Furthermore, we have challenged the diagnoses that are made at our catchment area hospital by inviting a Black Jamaican psychiatrist to re-evaluate routine diagnoses made at the Maudsley Hospital; this psychiatrist had previously reported that the rates of psychosis in Jamaica were similar to those among the White population in the UK (Hickling, 1991).

In the present study, we included all the in-patients on two wards, with a high proportion of patients from ethnic minority groups and from deprived inner-city areas . The Jamaican psychiatrist was asked to re-assess all consenting patients using his own clinical examination. There was no significant difference in the proportion of African–Caribbean patients that the Jamaican psychiatrist considered were suffering from psychosis or, more specifically, schizophrenia (44%) when his diagnoses were compared to those of the White UK psychiatrists (41%). Thus, misdiagnosis is unlikely to explain the increased incidence of psychosis in African–Caribbeans resident in the UK.

Migration

One of the earliest explanations offered to account for the increased incidence of psychosis among African–Caribbean people in the UK was that it was a product of the experience of migration (Sashidharan, 1993). An association between migration and mental illness was first established by Ödegaard's study in 1932, which showed that Norwegian immigrants in the USA had higher rates of schizophrenia than their compatriots who stayed in Norway (Ödegaard, 1932). It has been hypothesised that people with a high risk of psychosis are more likely to migrate (Ödegaard, 1932; Sashidharan, 1993), but there are problems in trying to equate the experience of Europeans migrating from one developed country to another with that of people moving from an underdeveloped country to a developed one. The theory does not take into consideration the underlying economic factors which led to migration in each group. This may have led to selection of a different subgroup of individuals (Sashidharan, 1993).

It has not been proved that there is a higher risk of development of schizophrenia in all immigrant groups. There are an equal number of studies showing higher rates of mental disorder in immigrants to those showing lower morbidity in immigrants (Canadian Task Force on Mental Health Issues Affecting Immigrants and Refugees, 1988); and although a recent study claimed that there was a high rate of schizophrenia in all ethnic minority groups in the UK (King *et al*, 1994), subsequent correspondence has questioned this (McKenzie, 1995*a*). There is little evidence for an increased risk of schizophrenia in the Asian population in the UK (Sashidharan, 1993; McKenzie, 1995*a*). Thus, it is likely that it is not migration itself but some factor in the UK which affects the African–Caribbean population leading to increased incidence of schizophrenia in this group.

Cannabis

Some consider that cannabis can be aetiologically important in the genesis of psychosis (Indian Hemp Drugs Commission, 1894; Andreasson *et al*, 1989; Thomas, 1993; Linszen *et al*, 1994). Cannabis can certainly cause a psychotic reaction, a type of toxic confusional state, and its use can lead to a relapse of psychosis (Thomas, 1993), but can it lead to a long-term psychosis and is it a particular risk factor in African–Caribbeans?

Andreasson *et al* (1989) showed that regular cannabis use before enlisting in the Swedish army doubled the risk of developing schizophrenia for subjects over the next 15 years. It is questionable whether greater cannabis use by people who later develop schizophrenia may be secondary to their premorbid personality abnormality. However, other researchers have claimed that cannabis may unmask psychotic symptoms in predisposed subjects (Breakey *et al*, 1974); people with psychosis who used cannabis before they became ill had an earlier age of onset of schizophrenia.

Even if regular cannabis use is a risk factor in schizophrenia, there is little evidence that cannabis use is higher among young African–Caribbeans in the UK than their White counterparts. In patients admitted to our own hospitals in south London, the same proportion of White and African–Caribbean patients admit to cannabis use (McKenzie *et al*, 1995*b*). Furthermore, though African–Caribbean patients were more likely to be urine-tested for cannabis, there were no differences in the proportions of patients who tested positive for cannabis (McGuire *et al*, 1994). If regular cannabis use is a risk factor for schizophrenia, there is no convincing evidence that it differentially affects African–Caribbean people rather than White people and so, by itself, it does not account for the increased incidence of schizophrenia in African–Caribbean people in the UK. The rates of psychosis in

Jamaica are not elevated, though the use of marijuana among working men in Jamaica is high, estimated at 40% (Dreher, 1982).

Genetics

There is a large genetic component to the risk of developing schizophrenia and other psychoses among White populations; up to 60–80% of the variance in liability may be due to genes (Kendler & Diehl, 1993). Though the lifetime risk of developing schizophrenia is 0.6–0.8%, this increases 10-fold among the siblings of people with schizophrenia, and is almost 50% for the identical twin of a person with schizophrenia. Therefore, the more genes that an individual shares with an affected person, the higher the risk of schizophrenia.

It has been argued that the increased risk of schizophrenia for African–Caribbean people in the UK may simply be due to an increased genetic risk. However, if African–Caribbean people have some particular genetic susceptibility to developing schizophrenia, then one would expect an increased incidence of schizophrenia in the Caribbean – there is no evidence of this. An incidence study in Jamaica reported rates for schizophrenia similar to those of the White population in the UK (Hickling & Rodgers-Johnson, 1995). Genetic hypotheses were also proffered for the increased incidence rate of psychosis in the African population living in the UK, but the African centre in the World Health Organization's International Pilot Study of Schizophrenia (Sartorius *et al*, 1986) did not find an increased incidence of schizophrenia. These findings confound arguments that there is a simple genetic explanation for the increased incidence of schizophrenia in African–Caribbean people in the UK.

However, investigations into the familial nature of schizophrenia have been useful in an unexpected way. In a small study, Sugarman & Craufurd (1994) examined the morbid risk for schizophrenia in the parents and siblings of people with schizophrenia and compared the risks for the relatives of White and African–Caribbean probands. They found that the morbid risk for developing schizophrenia in the parents of White patients was the same as in the parents of African–Caribbean patients. However, the morbid risk for the siblings of the African–Caribbean patients was much higher than that for the siblings of their White patients. The risk of developing schizophrenia was 16% for siblings of the African–Caribbean group while it was only 4% for the siblings of their White patients; among siblings of UK-born African–Caribbean probands the morbid risk was even higher at 27%.

Hutchinson *et al* (1996) have attempted to replicate this study. Once again, it was found that the morbid risk for schizophrenia for parents was the same in the two groups but that the morbid risk for siblings was increased in the African–Caribbean group, particularly for the siblings of patients who were born in the UK (morbid risk 26% for siblings of second-generation African–Caribbean patients, 4.3% for siblings of first-generation African–Caribbean patients, and 7% for siblings of White British patients).

The fact that, in these two studies, the parental morbid risk is the same for African–Caribbeans and Whites implies that the genetic risk is the same and that the increased morbid risk for siblings of the second-generation African–Caribbean patient group is not due to an increased genetic risk. Predisposing genes operate in both populations but other risk factors appear necessary in order for the vulnerability to be expressed as schizophrenia. Siblings have similar exposure to other risk factors and so the risk in the family is a function not only of the genetic risk but also of the environment to which family members are jointly exposed. The obvious conclusion to be drawn from these findings is that the increased incidence of schizophrenia in African–Caribbean people in the UK is due to an environmental effect operating preferentially in the UK on African–Caribbean people born in the UK.

Neurodevelopmental illness

Neurodevelopmental impairment is an important risk factor for schizophrenia in the White population. Much research suggests that schizophrenia can be a late consequence of aberrant brain development during foetal and neonatal life. Insults to the growing brain are thought to predispose the individual to later development of psychosis when the final maturational changes in brain organisation occur during adolescence and early adult life (Murray *et al*, 1992).

Obstetric complications and viral infections leading to brain injury are hypothesised as being important early environmental hazards (Murray *et al*, 1992; Sham *et al*, 1992; Gupta, 1993). White people with schizophrenia are more likely to have a history of obstetric complications than those who do not have a psychotic illness. This is particularly true for male patients with an early onset of illness. In addition, several studies suggested an increased incidence of schizophrenia in people who were in mid-gestation during the 1957 influenza epidemic (Sham *et al*, 1992). Are obstetric complications and prenatal viral infections more common or more significant in the African–Caribbean population in the UK, and could they explain the increased incidence of schizophrenia in this population?

The relationship between obstetric complications and ethnic groups is complex. The perinatal mortality rate in the Caribbean is four to five times that in the UK (World Health Organization, 1968), but there are no differences in the gestation-specific perinatal mortality rates between the offspring of African–Caribbean and European mothers in the UK (Lyon *et al*, 1994). A greater survival rate of low birth-weight African–Caribbean babies was reported in Birmingham (Eagles, 1991) and this could lead to more individuals with a history of perinatal brain trauma in the African–Caribbean population. However, recent evidence from a study of south London has shown an increase in perinatal mortality in African and African–Caribbean groups, mainly due to an increased number of women going into labour early and women suffering inter-uterine deaths (Lyon *et al*, 1994). It is therefore difficult to establish the overall effect of these different factors on the prevalence of obstetric complications or inter-uterine cerebral damage in the African and African–Caribbean populations in the UK.

We investigated whether obstetric complications were as common in African–Caribbean patients as they were in White patients using data from the Functional Psychosis Study (Harvey *et al*, 1990; Jones *et al*, 1993). This study concerns two consecutive samples of patients with psychosis admitted to two south London psychiatric hospitals. Sampling procedures were virtually identical. Patients were recruited if they had delusions, hallucinations or formal thought disorder in clear consciousness, as defined by the Research Diagnostic Criteria (Spitzer *et al*, 1978). Over 30% of the people in the sample were African–Caribbean, which allowed a comparison of the risk factors in the two groups (Harvey *et al*, 1990). Information on obstetric complications was collected by maternal interview.

We found that, though fewer African–Caribbean than White people with psychosis had a history of obstetric complications, there was no significant difference between the groups. We did not find any evidence that the higher incidence of psychosis in African–Caribbean people could be explained by an increase in obstetric complications.

Some researchers have hypothesised that the increased incidence may be due to infection of pregnant African–Caribbean women in the UK with viruses to which they do not have immunity (Gupta, 1993). Two viruses, in particular, have been suggested: influenza (Gupta, 1993) and rubella (Glover, 1989).

It is unlikely that the increased incidence of schizophrenia is due to differential exposure to influenza across the different ethnic groups. The 1957 influenza epidemic was global and reached the Caribbean at a similar time as it reached the UK. The infection rate was similar in the two countries (Spence *et al*, 1957; Duun, 1958), with reported preliminary findings suggesting an increase in births of African–Caribbean individuals who subsequently became psychotic after the 1957 influenza epidemic. However, in this small study there was no way of establishing whether the increase was any greater in the African–Caribbean than in the White population.

There was an epidemic of congenital rubella in the African–Caribbean population of the UK in the 1950s and 1960s. This occurred because rubella was not endemic in the Caribbean at that time, and so many of the women who migrated to the UK did not have immunological resistance to rubella (Glover, 1989). However, it is unlikely that the increased incidence of psychosis in the UK can be attributed to rubella-induced brain damage during pregnancy, since the increased incidence of psychosis is also reported in Africans in the UK (Wessely *et al*, 1991). The women brought up in Africa were exposed to rubella.

It is difficult to investigate obstetric complications or viral infections retrospectively. However, we can investigate the frequency of some outcomes of early cerebral insults, neurological disorders and brain abnormalities. If White and African–Caribbean people with psychoses have the same amount of neurodevelopmentally mediated disease, then it would be expected that those brain abnormalities which have been shown to be present in some White people with schizophrenia would be seen in a similar proportion of their African–Caribbean counterparts. No research has directly looked at brain structure but we have some evidence from the Functional Psychosis Study (Harvey *et al*, 1990; Jones *et al*, 1993) that African–Caribbean and White people with psychoses do have different risk-factor profiles for neurological disorders.

We looked at markers of neurological abnormality such as childhood central nervous system infections or epilepsy in people with psychoses and found that African–Caribbean people, as a group, had less evidence of neurological disorders than White people. This is contrary to expectations that increased incidence of schizophrenia in African–Caribbean people is due to excess exposure to maternal viral infection or obstetric complications.

Because there could be cultural differences in reporting both obstetric complications and neurological problems, we used the Functional Psychosis Study sample to look at the clinical hallmarks of neurologically mediated psychosis. People with neurologically mediated illnesses have an early onset of illness and problems with social adjustment. African–Caribbean people were less likely to have seen a psychiatrist for their illness before the age of 16 years. There were no differences in social adjustment.

Our findings indicate that an excess of neurodevelopmental illness does not explain the increased incidence of schizophrenia; there is no increase in obstetric complications, neurological disorders or the clinical hallmarks of neurologically mediated illness. Indeed, a lower proportion of African–Caribbean people with psychosis show evidence of neurodevelopmental illness.

An alternative approach

None of the hypotheses discussed above is able, on its own, to account for the increased incidence of psychosis in people of African–Caribbean origin living in the UK. However, our studies do suggest that the relative importance of certain risk factors may be different in African–Caribbean and White people with psychosis. Our family study (Hutchinson *et al*, 1996) and a study by Sugarman & Craufurd (1994) both point to an environmental risk factor operating on African–Caribbean individuals born in the UK. Research so far suggests that this is unlikely to be due to an excess of neurodevelopmentally mediated disease or cannabis consumption by African–Caribbean people.

Although misdiagnosis of psychosis is also an unlikely explanation, we do have evidence that some of the characteristics of illnesses in the two groups are different (McKenzie *et al*, 1995*c*). We followed-up African–Caribbean and White British patients who had entered the Functional Psychosis Study and who had a recent onset of illness; the average length of follow-up was four years. Members of the African–Caribbean group spent more time in a recovered state over the follow-up period, were less likely to have had a continuous illness and had more good outcomes from psychotic illnesses. Furthermore, the African–Caribbeans in the follow-up study were of a lower socio-economic status, and when this was taken into account the better outcome of the African–Caribbean patients became even more noticeable.

These findings raise questions about the type of psychosis to which African–Caribbean people living in the UK are especially susceptible. Bughra *et al* (1997) have shown, in a recent first-onset sample, that the increased incidence of schizophrenia in African–Caribbean people was due to an excess of schizophrenia which does not fall into the CATEGO category S+; that is, an increase in schizophrenia which does not have the core Schneiderian symptoms. Furthermore, there is evidence of an increased incidence of mania in African–Caribbean UK residents (Wessely *et al*, 1991; Van Os *et al*, 1994). Van Os *et al* (1996*a,b*) have shown that this increase is particularly marked in individuals with schizomanic psychoses. As mania can mimic schizophrenia, the increased rates of illness in African–Caribbean people could be due to an increase in psychoses which have a strong affective component.

Affective and schizoaffective psychoses are more frequently precipitated by life events than schizophrenia is (Bebbington *et al*, 1993).

Therefore, one explanation for the increased incidence of psychosis in African–Caribbean people in the UK could be an excess of psychotic illness mediated by social stress. Illnesses with an identifiable precipitant have a better prognosis than those due to constitutional factors in the individual (Vaillant, 1964; Van Os *et al*, 1994). Thus, the better prognosis for patients of Caribbean origin in our study may have been due to this group having more illness precipitated by social stress.

Such a hypothesis would explain the lower rate of neurological disorders in African–Caribbean people with psychoses; it would explain why the increase is in non-S+ schizophrenia, and it would explain why the familial risk in parents is similar whereas the risk for siblings of second-generation African–Caribbean people is increased. Therefore, social factors may be important risk-increasing factors in African–Caribbean people resident in the UK. One can only speculate on which social factors are involved. Material deprivation may well be important but, further than this, institutionalised racism and life events can lead to chronic stress (Perera *et al*, 1991).

The mechanism of action of these possible risk factors is not known. Research to date has tried to control for social class and other demographic factors when calculating rates (Van Os *et al*, 1996*a,b*) but it is difficult to know how the effects of multiple disadvantages interact with other risk factors, such as genetic predisposition. Any hypothesis based on the assumption that social stress is important will have to explain why the rates are not raised in the Asian population in the UK.

Investigation of the role of social factors and how they interact with known biological risk factors in the British African–Caribbean community is now well overdue. Establishing the role of such social factors would not only raise possibilities of prevention within the African–Caribbean community but could also provide an important pointer towards a possible causal role, rather than a precipitating role, for social factors in psychosis, a role that is currently discounted by much orthodox psychiatric research.

References

ANDREASSON, S., ALLBECK, P. & RYDBERG, U. (1989) Schizophrenia in users and non-users of cannabis: a longitudinal study. *Acta Psychiatrica Scandinavica*, **79**, 505–510.

BEBBINGTON, P., WILKINS, S., JONES, P., *et al* (1993) Life events and psychosis. Initial results from the Camberwell Collaborative Psychosis Study. *British Journal of Psychiatry*, **162**, 72–79.

BHUGRA, D., LEFF, J., MALLETT, R., *et al* (1997) Incidence and outcome of schizophrenia in Whites, African–Caribbeans and Asians in London. *Psychological Medicine*, **27**, 791–798.

BREAKEY, W. R., GOODELL, H., LORENZ, P. C., *et al* (1974) Hallucinogenic drugs as precipitants of schizophrenia. *Psychological Medicine*, **4**, 255–261.

CANADIAN TASK FORCE ON MENTAL HEALTH ISSUES AFFECTING IMMIGRANTS AND REFUGEES (1988) *Review of the Literature on Migrant Mental Health*. Ottawa: Ottawa Ministry Supply Services.

DREHER, M. C. (1982) *Working Men and Ganja in Jamaica. Marijuana Use in Rural Jamaica*. Philadelphia, PA: Philadelphia Institute of Study of Human Issues.

DUUN, F. L. (1958) Pandemic influenza in 1957: review of international spread of New Asian strain. *Journal of the American Medical Association*, **166**, 1140–1148.

EAGLES, J. M. (1991) The relationship between schizophrenia and immigration. Are there alternatives to psychosocial hypotheses? *British Journal of Psychiatry*, **159**, 783–789.

FERNANDO, S. (1988) *Race and Culture in Psychiatry*. London: Croom Helm.

GLOVER, G. R. (1989) Why is there an increased rate of schizophrenia in British Caribbeans? *British Journal of Hospital Medicine*, **42**, 48–51.

GUPTA, S. (1993) Can environmental factors explain the epidemiology of schizophrenia in immigrant groups? *Social Psychiatry and Epidemiology*, **28**, 263–266.

HARRISON, G., OWENS, D., HOLTON, A., *et al* (1988) A prospective study of severe mental disorder in African–Caribbean patients. *Psychological Medicine*, **18**, 643–657.

HARVEY, I., WILLIAMS, M., MCGUFFIN, P., *et al* (1990) The functional psychoses in African–Caribbeans. *British Journal of Psychiatry*, **157**, 515–522.

HICKLING, F. W. (1991) Psychiatric admission rates in Jamaica, 1971 and 1988. *British Journal of Psychiatry*, **159**, 817–821.

—— & RODGERS-JOHNSON, P. (1995) The incidence of first-contact schizophrenia in Jamaica. *British Journal of Psychiatry*, **167**, 193–196.

HUTCHINSON, G., TAKEI, N., FAHY, T., *et al* (1996) Morbid risk for schizophrenia in the parents and siblings of African–Caribbean and White probands. *British Journal of Psychiatry*, **169**, 776–780.

INDIAN HEMP DRUGS COMMISSION (1894) *Report of the Indian Hemp Drugs Commission, 1893–1894*. Simla, India: Government Printing Office.

JONES, P. B., BEBBINGTON, P., FOERSTER, A., *et al* (1993) Premorbid social underachievement in schizophrenia. Results from the Camberwell Collaborative Psychosis study. *British Journal of Psychiatry*, **162**, 65–71.

KENDLER, K. S. & DIEHL, S. R. (1993) Genetics of schizophrenia: a current, genetic–epidemiological perspective. *Schizophrenia Bulletin*, **19**, 261–285.

KING, M., COKER, E., LEAVEY, G., *et al* (1994) Incidence of psychotic illness in London: a comparison of ethnic groups. *British Medical Journal*, **309**, 1115–1119.

LEFF, J., FISHER, M. & BERTELSEN, A. (1976) A cross-national study of mania. *British Journal of Psychiatry*, **129**, 428–442.

LEWIS, G., CROFT-JEFFREYS, C. & DAVID, A. (1990) Are British psychiatrists racist? *British Journal of Psychiatry*, **157**, 410–415.

LINSZEN, D. H., DINGEMANS, P. M. & LENOIR, M. E. (1994) Cannabis and the course of psychotic illness. *Archives of General Psychiatry*, **51**, 273–279.

LITTLEWOOD, R. & LIPSEDGE, M. (1981) Some social and phenomenological characteristics of psychotic immigrants. *Psychological Medicine*, **11**, 289–302

LYON, A. J., CARKSON, P., JEFFREY, I., *et al* (1994) Effect of ethnic origin of mother on fetal outcome. *Archives of Disease in Childhood*, **70**, 40–43.

MCGUIRE, P., JONES, P., HARVEY, I., *et al* (1994) Cannabis and acute psychosis. *Schizophrenia Research*, **13**, 161–168.

MCKENZIE, K. J. (1995*a*) Psychotic illness in ethnic groups: accuracy of variables describing ethnic minority groups is important. *British Medical Journal*, **310**, 333.

——, MURRAY, R., JONES, P., *et al* (1995*b*) Aetiology of schizophrenia in African–Caribbeans. *Schizophrenia Research*, **15**, 194–195.

——, VAN OS, J., FAHY, T., *et al* (1995*c*) Psychosis with good prognosis in Afro-Caribbean people now living in the United Kingdom. *British Medical Journal*, **311**, 1325–1327.

MURRAY, R. M., O'CALLAGHAN, E., CASTLE, D. J., *et al* (1992) Neurodevelopmental approach to the classification of schizophrenia. *Schizophrenia Bulletin,* **18**, 319–332.

ÖDEGAARD, O. (1932) Emigration and insanity: a study of mental disease among Norwegian-born population in Minnesota. *Acta Psychiatrica et Neurologica Scandinavia Supplementum,* **4**, 1–26.

PERERA, R., OWENS, D. G. C. & JOHNSTONE, E. (1991) Disabilities and circumstances of schizophrenic patients – a follow-up study. VII: Ethnic aspects. A comparison of three matched groups. *British Journal of Psychiatry,* **159** (suppl. 13), 40–42.

ROBINS, E. & GUZE, S. B. (1970) Establishment of diagnostic validity in psychiatric illness: its application to schizophrenia. *American Journal of Psychiatry,* **126**, 983–987.

SARTORIUS, N., JABLENSKY, A., KORTEN, A., *et al* (1986) Early manifestations and first contact incidence of schizophrenia in different cultures. *Psychological Medicine,* **16**, 909–928.

SASHIDHARAN, S. P. (1993) African–Caribbeans and schizophrenia: the ethnic vulnerability hypothesis re-examined. *International Review of Psychiatry,* **5**, 129–144.

SHAM, P. C., O'CALLAGHAN, E., TAKEI, N., *et al* (1992) Schizophrenia following pre-natal exposure to influenza epidemics between 1939 and 1960. *British Journal of Psychiatry,* **160**, 461–466.

SPENCE, L., ANDERSON, R. & DOWNS, W. G. (1957) The isolation of influenza virus during an epidemic in Trinidad, British West Indies. *Caribbean Medical Journal,* **19**, 174–178.

SPITZER, R. L., ENDICOTT, J. & ROBINS, E. (1978) *Research Diagnostic Criteria (RDC) for a Selected Group of Functional Disorders* (3rd edn). New York: New York State Psychiatric Institute.

SUGARMAN, P. A. & CRAUFURD, D. (1994) Schizophrenia in the African–Caribbean community. *British Journal of Psychiatry,* **164**, 474–480.

THOMAS, H. (1993) Psychiatric symptoms in cannabis users. *British Journal of Psychiatry,* **163**, 141–149.

VAILLANT, G. E. (1964) Prospective prediction of schizophrenic remission. *Archives of General Psychiatry,* **11**, 509–518.

VAN OS, J., FAHY, T., BEBBINGTON, P., *et al* (1994) The influence of life events on the subsequent course of psychotic illness. *Psychological Medicine,* **24**, 503–513.

——, CASTLE, D., TAKEI, N., *et al* (1996a) Schizophrenia in ethnic minorities: clarification from the 1991 census. *Psychological Medicine,* **26**, 203–208.

——, TAKEI, N., CASTLE, D., *et al* (1996b) The incidence of mania: time trends in relation to gender and ethnicity. *Social Psychiatry and Psychiatric Epidemiology,* **3**, 129–136.

WESSELY, S., CASTLE, D., DER, G., *et al* (1991) Schizophrenia and African–Caribbeans: a case control study. *British Journal of Psychiatry,* **159**, 795–801.

WORLD HEALTH ORGANIZATION (1968) *Deliveries and Complications of Pregnancy, Childbirth and the Puerperium.* World Health Organization Statistics Report 21, 468–471.

7 Common mental disorders among African–Caribbean general practice attenders in Brixton, London

KEITH LLOYD and LYNN St LOUIS

Depression and anxiety are by far the most common mental disorders seen in primary care settings. Less than 6% of people with mental health problems seen in primary care settings are referred to secondary care services. Less than 10% of general practice psychiatry involves people with psychotic mental illnesses such as schizophrenia. However, most attention about ethnicity and mental health has focused on secondary care and psychosis. There has been almost no work looking specifically at the primary care management and natural history of non-psychotic disorders such as depression and anxiety among African–Caribbean people in this country (Lloyd & St Louis, 1993; see Chapter 19 for Asian samples).

We use the term Black to describe African–Caribbean people born in the West Indies or sub-Saharan Africa, or those people born in this country who consider themselves to be ethnically West Indian or African. The authors we have quoted use a variety of different conventions which will be made explicit as appropriate.

Attendance rates and presenting complaints

About 98% of the general population in the UK is registered with a general practitioner (GP) and it seems likely that a similar proportion applies for the African–Caribbean population, most of whom live in urban areas (Giggs, 1986; Johnson, 1986).

The earliest studies of psychiatric morbidity among Black primary care attenders were carried out among first-generation migrants from the Caribbean to Birmingham (Pinsent, 1963) and Brixton, London (Kiev, 1965). Both studies reported higher overall consultation rates for Black people of Jamaican origin compared with White people of British origin. However, Pinsent found that Jamaican attenders were less likely than British attenders to have a psychiatric disorder, whereas Kiev reported the opposite.

More recent studies have not shown higher consultation rates among Black patients for psychiatric problems, of either gender, compared with White British patients. Gillam *et al* (1989) studied over 67 000 general practice consultations in Brent, North London, over a one-year period. Ethnicity was defined using a composite of "race and nationality". It was found that White British patients consulted more than any other ethnic group for GP-defined psychological problems. Consultation rates for psychiatric problems were lowest in West Indian and Asian women. Although consultation rates were standardised for age and gender, they were not adjusted for socio-economic status. Regardless of the reason for consulting, White British patients were more likely than any other group to leave the surgery with a follow-up appointment, a prescription or a certificate.

Symptom detection and recognition

GPs detect about 60% of the psychological problems in the people they see (Goldberg & Huxley, 1992; also discussed in Chapters 3 and 4). Any symptom can have a range of different implications for the patient and the GP in different cultural and interpersonal settings (Helman, 1990). Culture, class and gender all play a part, as do time constraints and many other structural and process issues.

Short screening questionnaires have been advocated as one way of improving detection and recognition of mental disorders in primary care (Lloyd & Jenkins, 1994). Shapiro *et al* (1987) administered the General Health Questionnaire (GHQ; Goldberg, 1972) to primary care attenders in North America and reported a "marked increase in detection of psychiatric morbidity among the elderly, Blacks and men". The GHQ is used commonly as a 'gold standard' for detecting psychiatric morbidity in patient populations and it has been validated in a wide range of settings. It cannot be ruled out that use of the GHQ among this group leads to a distorted picture of 'true' morbidity. Whether the bias is towards over- or under-reporting of cases is not known. There may be problems associated with the application and translation of European disease categories and concepts to settings other than those from which the categories evolved

(Kleinman, 1987). Categories, concepts and symptoms which have coherence in one cultural setting may lack meaning or have different implications in another cultural context.

A different approach is to ask the patients themselves why they have attended the GP. Balarajan *et al* (1989) performed a community survey of 63 966 people. They asked about consultation behaviour over the preceding 14 days. After adjustment for age, gender and socio-economic group they derived odds ratios for consultation by ethnic group. Consultation for all disorders, among adults aged 16–65 years, was highest for men and women of Pakistani origin. Significantly more consultations were also seen for men of West Indian and Indian origin than among White patients. West Indian and Indian women did not consult significantly more than White women (for details of a community survey see Chapter 23).

Factors influencing consulting behaviour for common psychiatric disorders

Consultation behaviour is influenced by the severity of the problem, the individual's propensity to seek help, the accessibility of services and the availability of alternative resources (Dressler & Badger, 1985; Williams *et al*, 1990). It is not known for certain whether African–Caribbean patients are more or less likely than White patients to seek help for psychiatric disorders.

Kiev (1965) raised the possibility that Black patients were more likely than White British patients to seek help from alternative and traditional sources rather than medical practitioners. However, medical pluralism is probably as much a feature of White British culture as it is of Black cultures (Helman, 1990).

Factors such as cultural and personal attitudes to health and health care, distrust of the health care system by ethnic minorities, lifestyle and language barriers, lack of understanding and tolerance shown by health care professionals and social and psychological stresses associated with discrimination have all been implicated as influences on help-seeking behaviour (Rathwell, 1984; Gillam, 1990). Discrimination and overt and institutional racism are frequently discussed in relation to hospital and community treatment of major mental illness among African–Caribbean people (Littlewood & Lipsedge, 1988; Francis *et al*, 1989). Racist views held by hospital and primary care workers are only one aspect of the problem. Beyond this, in areas such as mental health, Black people are faced with institutional racism which treats their beliefs, values and experiences as inferior, bizarre or deviant and as a result they find themselves subjected to poor or more brutal psychiatric treatment (Lloyd & Moodley, 1992). There is also a problem with the stigma attached to mental illness and, more fundamentally, with differing models of mental illness (also see Chapter 4). Effective interventions exist for well-recognised and operationally defined conditions such as major depression.

Methods

A key study to investigate rates of common mental disorders in a south London general practice was set up. The aims of the study were to investigate over 12 months the symptom profiles, service utilisation, attitudes, treatment and clinical and social outcomes of common mental disorders among African–Caribbean general practice attenders and compared with matched White British attenders. The study was conducted in a group general practice in Brixton with five partners: two male, three female; all White and of middle-class British backgrounds. About 40% of the patients registered with this practice were of African–Caribbean origin. Consent was sought from all attenders to complete the 12-item GHQ (Goldberg & Williams, 1988). Goldberg & Williams (1988) discuss the cross-cultural validity of the questionnaire, which was originally developed in London. A threshold of 2 was used to identify possible distress. The questionnaires were distributed in the waiting room by L. St L. (who is a Black British woman). Large-print versions and assistance were available for people who had difficulty completing the questionnaire.

A subsample of Black and White attenders were asked whether they would mind being interviewed at home. Those giving informed consent were administered the Clinical Interview Schedule (CIS; Lewis *et al*, 1992), the Social Supports and Stresses Interview (Jenkins *et al*, 1981) and the Short Explanatory Model Interview (SEMI) devised by the authors and based on the work of Kleinman (1980; Lloyd *et al*, 1998).

The CIS is a structured interview to elicit the type and severity of psychological symptoms and to permit a diagnosis to be made according to the ICD–10 produced by the World Health Organization (1992). The SEMI is a semi-structured questionnaire that is amenable to either qualitative or quantitative analysis and allows the user's perspective to be recorded. The GP recorded details about the consultation on a standard form. Subsequent attendances and other help-seeking visits were reviewed over the next 12 months. After this, the patients were re-interviewed.

Results

Black men were very under-represented among surgery attenders. Indeed, very few of those who did attend gave consent to participate in the study. This left a very unrepresentative sample of men who participated fully in the study. Further studies have taken place to explore the reasons for this and will be presented elsewhere. The results presented here are for the 304 female attenders recruited into the study.

Demographic characteristics

The ethnic diversity of the women interviewed was not reflected by the 1991 census categories (see Table 1). For example, within the White category there were English, Scottish, Welsh, Irish, French, Californian and Australian women. Many of the women who classified themselves as 'Black other' when forced to choose a census category were younger Black women born in the UK. At a later interview more detailed information was collected about self-definition of ethnicity and class. The mean age of the whole sample was 34 years. There were no significant differences between mean ages of women by census ethnic classification. However, the ages of Black Caribbean women followed a bimodal distribution, with one peak reflecting elders who were first-generation migrants and the other peak reflecting younger Black British women. Overall, 48% of the sample worked outside the home. There were differences by census ethnic group in the proportions of women who described themselves as doing manual work: 66% of Black African women, 70% of Black Caribbean women, 46% of Black other women and 43% of White women.

Psychiatric, general practice and users' views of distress

Of the women assessed, 154 scored two or more on the 12-item GHQ indicating probable psychological distress to a psychiatrist. There were

TABLE 1
Ethnicity of sample by 1991 census categories

Census category	n
Black African	30
Black Caribbean	37
Black other	76
White	150

TABLE 2
Mean scores on the 12-item General Health Questionnaire for respondents with psychological distress

Ethnicity	Mean	95% CI
Black	5.681	5.02–6.34
Non-Black	5.658	5.25–6.06
Black British	5.24	4.28–6.17
Black Caribbean	4.88	3.6–16.15
Black African	8.42	6.66–10.18*

* ANOVA $F=2.818$, $P=0.028$.

no differences between Black and White women in terms of mean GHQ score. However, there was significant intra-ethnic variations: Black African women had significantly higher GHQ scores (Table 2). There were few inter-ethnic differences in CIS symptom profiles. There were no differences in somatic symptoms, which were 50% in Black people and 52% in non-Black people. The only significant differences were for poor concentration and forgetfulness and anxiety, both being reported less frequently by Black respondents (odds ratios 0.72 (0.12–0.98) and 0.29 (0.11–0.71)).

The GPs had a different perspective. They recorded physical problems in 83% of Black and 86% of White women who were GHQ positive, but noted a psychiatric problem in 26% of the Black and 34% of the White GHQ-positive women (Table 3). They noted a social problem in about 30% of the women. To investigate further this discrepancy, patients' own accounts of their problems were elicited.

Black and White women gave broadly similar explanations. The categories that arose naturally from the data are shown in Table 4. The people who were GHQ cases felt that they had visited a doctor because of a physical problem. Non-specific explanations such as, " I feel tired, I have no energy" were also stated frequently as a reason for consulting. Psychological reasons for consulting came quite a long way down the list. Overall, the women were more likely to agree with the GPs' diagnoses than with the psychiatric rating scales.

Expectations and service delivery

Black women were less likely than non-Black women to say they knew what they wanted from the doctor and less likely to say they wanted a clear explanation of their symptoms (odds ratio 0.25 (0.11–0.50)). Similarly, they were much less likely to make multiple requests of their doctors (odds ratio 0.23 (0.1–0.49)).

TABLE 3

General practitioners' views of presenting problems among General Health Questionnaire-positive attenders

Presenting problem	Black (%)	Non-Black (%)
Physical illness	83	86
Psychiatric illness	26	34
Social problem	32	36

Over the subsequent 12 months the GPs offered a variety of treatments. Most people were prescribed medication of some sort. A few received an antidepressant, fewer still received a hypnotic or anxiolytic. A few patients were referred to other agencies for either physical treatments or for counselling or psychotherapy. While none of the White patients referred themselves to accident and emergency during the follow-up year, four (5%) of the Black patients did so, which is significant on Fisher's Exact Test ($P=0.01$).

Women were higher than average general practice attenders. They consulted frequently over the 12-month follow-up with a mean of over 10 visits per year. The average number of visits per year in UK primary care (varying with age) is between 3 and 5. Black African women consulted significantly less often than any other group (mean 4.9 visits per year, ANOVA $F=5.07$, $P=0.00098$).

Outcomes and satisfaction

At 12-month follow-up the mean GHQ score for Black African women was 2, for Black Caribbean women 2.8, Black British women 3.1 and

TABLE 4

Service users' views of presenting problem among General Health Questionnaire-positive attenders

Presenting problem	Black (%)	Non-Black (%)
Physical	52	63
Non-specific	23	18
Psychological	15	20
Marital/family	3	0
Administrative	19	27
Child	16	10
Other	2	1
No reason	11	3

White women 3.3. All groups had improved, but had not recovered completely.

Subjects were asked what they thought about the care they received from their GP. Black women were significantly more likely to say they were dissatisfied with the care they received (although the figure was not as significant as the expected value of 21%; Table 5). Black African women patients were the least satisfied; they were the group who were most distressed at outset and attended least frequently.

Discussion

Above all, it must be emphasised that this was a small study in one area of London. The extent to which results can be generalised is not clear.

Arguably the most striking feature of this study might be the failure to engage Black men. This partly reflects their low utilisation of primary care but may also be due to the fact that the interviewers were all female, since we had matched for ethnicity but not gender.

In terms of symptom profiles and severity there were few inter-ethnic differences but there were some intra-ethnic differences. Black African women appeared to be more distressed on the GHQ. They did not, however, report more psychological distress. There were no ethnic differences in GP diagnoses. The doctors made a psychiatric diagnosis in about 30% of GHQ-positive patients. This may be low because we used a low caseness threshold. Interestingly, the women agreed more with the GP diagnoses than they did with the psychiatric rating scales. There were no ethnic differences in treatment. Black respondents were more likely to refer themselves to accident and emergency departments.

There were few inter-ethnic differences in service utilisation, but Black African women attended significantly less often – no more often than the national average for all patients. This may reflect the fact that

TABLE 5
Dissatisfaction with care received by General Health Questionnaire-positive GP attenders

Ethnicity	% not satisfied	Odds ratio	95% CI
Black	21	4.01	1.4–12.0
Non-Black	7		NS
Black African	23		NS
Black Caribbean	16		NS
Black other	15		NS

they got better: all the subjects' GHQ scores improved over the 12-month follow-up. White patients expected more from their GPs. Black patients were significantly less satisfied with the service they received. No study to date has compared users' reasons for consulting with the GP's assessment and that of a psychiatric screening questionnaire. It may be that GPs are not recognising psychiatric morbidity in African–Caribbean patients, it may be that patients are not telling the GPs about their psychosocial problems, or that African–Caribbean patients experience less psychiatric morbidity than White British patients. There have not been any studies that have fully controlled for social class or gender. Medical researchers have, by and large, been reluctant to address issues of discrimination. Additionally, no study has used research instruments specifically designed for use with African–Caribbean patients and few attempts have been made to validate existing instruments in this group.

Effective service planning and delivery depend on the availability of accurate and appropriate data. Such data are only just beginning to be collected. Service developments should be evidence-based where possible and presented in a form that will influence policy makers and purchasers.

Acknowledgements

K. L. was supported by the Leverhulme Trust. We thank A. H. Mann and K. S. Jacob for their support and encouragement.

References

BALARAJAN, R., YUEN, P. & SONI RALEIGH, V. (1989) Ethnic differences in general practitioner consultations. *British Medical Journal*, 299, 958–968.

DRESSLER, W. W. & BADGER, L. W. (1985) Epidemiology of depressive symptoms in black communities. *Journal of Nervous & Mental Diseases*, 173, 212–220.

FRANCIS, E., DAVID, J. & JOHNSON, N. (1989) Black people and psychiatry in the UK. An alternative to institutional care. *Psychiatric Bulletin*, 13, 482–485.

GIGGS, J. (1986) Ethnic status and mental illness in urban areas. In *Health, Race & Ethnicity* (eds D. Phillips & T. Rathwell), pp. 137–174. London: Croom Helm.

GILLAM, S. (1990) Ethnicity and the use of health services. *Postgraduate Medical Journal*, 66, 989–993.

——, JARMAN, B., WHITE, P., *et al* (1989) Ethnic differences in consultation rates in urban general practice. *British Medical Journal*, 299, 953–957.

GOLDBERG, D. (1972) *The Detection of Psychiatric Illness by Questionnaire* (GHQ). Maudsley Monograph 21. Oxford: Oxford University Press.

—— & WILLIAMS, P. (1988) *A User's Guide to the General Health Questionnaire*. Windsor: NFER–Nelson.

—— & HUXLEY, P. (1992) *Common Mental Disorders: A Bio-Social Model*. London: Routledge.

HELMAN, C. G. (1990) *Culture, Health & Illness* (2nd edn). Bristol: Wright.

JENKINS, R., MANN, A. H. & BELSEY, E. (1981) The background, design and use of a short interview to assess social stress and support in research and clinical settings. *Social Science & Medicine,* **15,** 195–203.

JOHNSON, M. (1986) Inner city residents, ethnic minorities and primary health care in the West Midlands. In *Health, Race and Ethnicity* (eds D. Phillips & T. Rathwell), pp. 192–212. London: Croom Helm.

KIEV, A. (1965) Psychiatric morbidity of West Indian immigrants in an urban group practice. *British Journal of Psychiatry,* **111,** 51–56.

KLEINMAN, A. (1980) *Patients and Healers in the Context of Culture,* pp. 138–145. Berkley, CA: University of California Press.

—— (1987) Anthropology and psychiatry: the role of culture in cross-cultural research on illness. *British Journal of Psychiatry,* **151,** 447–454.

LEWIS, G., PELOSI, A., ARAYA, R., *et al* (1992) Measuring psychiatric disorder in the community: a standardized assessment for use by lay interviewers. *Psychological Medicine,* **22,** 465–486.

LITTLEWOOD, R. & LIPSEDGE, M. (1988) Psychiatric illness among British Afro-Caribbeans. *British Medical Journal,* **296,** 950–951.

LLOYD, K. & MOODLEY, P. (1992) Psychotropic medication and ethnicity: an in-patient survey. *Social Psychiatry & Psychiatric Epidemiology,* **27,** 95–101.

—— & ST LOUIS, L. (1993) Depression and anxiety among Afro-Caribbean general practice attenders in Britain. *International Journal of Social Psychiatry,* **39,** 1–9.

—— & JENKINS, R. (1994) Prevention in medical settings: primary care. In *Prevention in Psychiatry* (eds E. Paykel & R. Jenkins), pp. 198–209. London: Gaskell.

——, Jacob, K., Patel, V., *et al* (1998) The development and use of the Short Explanatory Model Interview. *Psychological Medicine,* **28,** 1231–1237.

PINSENT, R. (1963) Morbidity in an immigrant population. *Lancet, ii,* 437–438.

RATHWELL,T.(1984) General practice, ethnicity & health service delivery. *Social Science and Medicine,* **19,** 123–130.

SHAPIRO, S., GERMAN, P., SKINNER, E., *et al* (1987) An experiment to change detection & management of mental morbidity in primary care. *Medical Care,* **25,** 327–329.

WILLIAMS, P., WILKINSON, G. & ARREGHINI, E. (1990) The determinants of help seeking for psychological distress in primary health care settings. In *Psychological Disorders in General Medical Settings* (eds N. Sartorius & D. Goldberg), pp. 21–33. Toronto: Hogrefe & Huber.

WORLD HEALTH ORGANIZATION (1992) *Tenth Revision of the International Classification of Diseases and Related Health Problems* (ICD–10). Geneva: WHO.

8 Ethnicity, drinking patterns and alcohol-related problems in England

RAYMOND COCHRANE

While there has been considerable research (and speculation) about the extent of mental health problems among the non-White minority ethnic groups in Britain (those of south Asian and African–Caribbean origin), there has been relatively little attention given to the way in which these groups engage with alcohol, or the extent of alcohol-related problems.

Some significant findings emerged from an analysis of mental hospital admissions in England when these data were broken down by diagnosis and country of birth (Cochrane & Bal, 1989) (see Table 1):

(a) The rate of mental hospital admissions for alcohol-related diagnoses for men born in India but living in England was considerably in excess of the native-born rate (and had shown a much greater rate of increase over the preceding decade).

(b) Men born in Pakistan had a negligible rate of in-patient admissions for alcohol problems, and the rate had declined between 1971 and 1981.

(c) Men born in the Caribbean had conspicuously lower rates of treatment for alcohol problems than native-born men.

(d) Women migrants to England had consistently lower rates than native-born women.

Of course, treatment-based data do not reveal the true prevalence with any reliability, as only an uncertain fraction of people with alcohol-related problems will find their way into formal psychiatric care (also discussed in Chapter 5). In addition, it is important to note that the figures for hospital admissions refer to country of birth not ethnic origin. While it is unlikely that the Caribbean-born group will contain many White people, the Indian-born group may well contain people of British

TABLE 1
Age-adjusted rates of mental hospital in-patient admissions for alcohol-related disorders[1] in England, 1981

Country of birth	Rate per 100 000	
	Males	Females
England	49	22
West Indies	26	10
India	75	7
Pakistan [2]	6	1 [3]

1. ICD–9 codes 291 and 303.
2. Includes Bangladesh.
3. One case only.

descent and the UK-born patients will include a number of African–Caribbean, south Asian and other minority ethnic group members.

McKeigue & Karmi (1993) have examined all the reliable evidence available concerning levels of alcohol consumption and alcohol-related problems in the largest minority ethnic groups in the UK (except the Irish). They examined data from community surveys and hospital admissions, as well as alcohol-related mortality rates. Their analysis of data on mortality from causes likely to be alcohol-related between 1979 and 1983 showed that Caribbean-born men and women had a lower rate of deaths from chronic liver disease and cirrhosis of the liver than did the whole population (standard mortality ratios 91 and 52 for men and women, respectively) while south Asian male immigrants had conspicuously higher rates (2.5 times greater than the national average).

Balarajan & Yuen (1986) examined General Household Survey figures and found that African–Caribbean people consumed less alcohol, and were less likely to be heavy drinkers than White people, a finding confirmed in several other studies. A similar pattern of relatively light drinking was found by McKeigue & Karmi (1993) when they examined the data available from community surveys of drinking patterns among Asian men and women.

McKeigue & Karmi were able to conclude the part of their review relating to Britain's Black population by stating that:

"rates of heavy drinking and alcohol-related problems (appear) to be about 50% lower in African–Caribbean men and women than in the native British population".

They reached no conclusion about what average drinking levels were, or any differences between those of African–Caribbean origin born in the West Indies and those born in Britain. With respect to the south Asian population, they concluded that average consumption levels were relatively low among Gujarati Hindus, Muslims and all Asian women, but that heavy drinking was not uncommon in Sikh men. However, male Sikh drinking levels were probably no higher than the levels found in White men, but their alcohol-related psychiatric admissions were conspicuously higher.

> "The association between average alcohol consumption and rates of alcohol-related morbidity, though valid across other minority groups, appears therefore not to hold for Sikh men" (McKeigue & Karmi, 1993).

The study

The study reported here had five main aims:

(a) To compare the pattern of alcohol use in minority ethnic groups with that found in the native White population.
(b) To determine the level of alcohol-related problems in the main (non-White) minority ethnic groups in England.
(c) To assess the trends in drinking patterns across generations.
(d) To discover whether the factors that are known to be associated with heavier drinking in the majority White population are also predictive of heavier drinking in minority groups, and to assess whether the differential distribution of these variables between ethnic groups could account for differences in drinking patterns found.
(e) So far as possible, to relate drinking habits to religious/cultural factors.

Because the limited data available indicated that few significant alcohol-related problems existed in minority ethnic women, only men were included in these studies. Although Hindu and Muslim men were included in the original study, only data for Sikh men (together with Black and White men) are reported here. Details of drinking patterns for other groups can be found in Cochrane & Bal (1990).

Terminology

In this chapter the ethnic classification of respondents uses the terms Sikh, Black and White. Sikhs defined themselves by their religious affiliation and the place of origin of their ancestors (the Punjab). The Black group had to be of self-defined African–Caribbean origin (not African). One man who defined himself as White but was considered to be Black by the (Black) interviewer was excluded. The term White was preferred for the native UK-born ethnically English comparison group, rather than English, because, although all the respondents in this group had been born in England (not Scotland, Ireland or Wales), so were many of the Sikh and Black respondents.

Method

To recruit a sample of 200 White UK-born, 200 Black and 200 Sikh men the names of men between the ages of 17 and 65 years were selected at random from the lists of eight general practices in the West Midlands. Practices were selected on the basis of location, so that those in areas with large Asian and Black populations, as well as those with fewer minority ethnic residents, were included in the survey. Details of how ethnic origin was identified and other methodological points are reported in Cochrane & Bal (1990) and Cochrane & Howell (1995).

The men selected were sent a letter, signed by their general practioner (GP), explaining in general terms the purpose and nature of the project. The rights of respondents to refuse, and the confidentiality of their responses, were stressed. The letters were translated into appropriate Asian languages and explained that interviews would be carried out at home, in the mother-tongue of the interviewee, and by interviewers of the same ethno-cultural background as the interviewees.

Interviewers were required to make three attempts to contact each respondent and a proportion of the work of each interviewer was back-checked, either by a second personal visit to the respondents by a supervisor, or by a telephone call.

The questionnaire used in the study was based on that used in the World Health Organizion's Three Centre Survey (Rootman & Moser, 1984). The central part was a retrospective drinking diary covering the week prior to interview. For each day in the previous week respondents were questioned about the number of occasions on which they had taken alcohol, how much, what kind of drinks were consumed and where and with whom they had been drinking. Other sections of the questionnaire covered reasons for drinking and for not drinking, problems stemming from alcohol use, a mental health scale and a range of demographic variables.

Results

Table 2 summarises the data obtained from the survey which relates to the drinking habits of the three groups of men. We adopted the standard conversion formula of one half-pint of beer, one glass of wine or one pub measure of spirits equating to one unit of alcohol. Sikhs were the most frequent drinkers with 41% drinking on at least three occasions in the week prior to interview, while less than half this proportion of Black men reported this frequency of drinking. On the other hand the Sikh group also contained the highest proportion (27.5%) of complete abstainers. The modal pattern for the White and Black groups was occasional (once or twice per week) drinking. Because they were the most frequent drinkers, the Sikh men also reported consuming the largest quantity of alcohol on average and the Black men by far the least. However, when only regular drinkers were considered the Sikh and White group had almost identical averages of 25 units per week. Even among the regular drinkers, Black men consumed less alcohol, on average, than their White and Sikh counterparts.

More data on the pattern of drinking reported by men from these three ethnic groups can be found in Table 3. Beer was overwhelmingly the preferred drink in all three groups, accounting for between 77% and 90% of the previous week's consumption. A significant quantity of spirits was consumed by the Black sample (one datum, which raises some methodological questions addressed later). Most Sikh men drank in pubs and very few in clubs, which were used more frequently by the Black and White samples. In all three groups about one-third of the alcohol taken was consumed at home.

Lone drinking was infrequent among White men but not uncommon in Sikhs and Black men. White men were also substantially more likely to drink with their families than the other two groups (even though they were less likely to be married than Sikh men).

The questionnaire used for surveying the extent of alcohol-related problems contained various relevant questions as well as an 11-item Alcohol Problems Scale. This unstandardised scale included items

TABLE 2
Drinking patterns in three ethnic groups

Variable	White	Black	Sikh
Regular drinkers[1] (%)	35.5	16.5	41.0
Occasional drinkers (%)	57.5	63.5	31.5
Abstainers[2] (%)	7.0	20.0	27.5
Mean units of alcohol per week			
All drinkers	14.6	7.9	17.3
Regular drinkers	25.2	19.0	25.4

1. At least three times a week.
2. No alcohol taken in previous year.

TABLE 3
Drinking patterns in three ethnic groups

	Percentage of total week's drinking		
	White	Black	Sikh
Drink (units)			
Beer	89	77	90
Wine	6	7	2
Spirits	5	16	8
Where (occasions)			
Pub	55	43	61
Club	24	20	3
Home	15	30	31
Elsewhere	6	7	4
Who with (occasions)[1]			
Alone	6	25	24
Friends/workmates	62	40	51
Family	42	28	26

1. These percentages do not add to 100% as on some occasions drinking took place with both friends and family.

about personal and social problems which may be related to alcohol misuse, but was not an alcohol dependency screening scale. An arbitrary threshold score of four was used to identify those with significant problems related to their alcohol consumption. Table 4 summarises all the data relevant to the second research aim (to uncover the level of alcohol-related problems in the ethnic minority groups surveyed).

About one-quarter of all the Sikh and White men interviewed reported drinking more than the recommended safe level of alcohol

TABLE 4
Alcohol-related problems in three ethnic groups

Variable	White (%)	Black (%)	Sikh (%)
Drinking more than 20 units	24.5	8.0	27.0
Drunk at least once a week	9.0	0.0	10.0
Drunk occasionally	32.5	7.5	30.5
Felt should reduce consumption	34.5	22.5	39.5
Medical advice to stop drinking	7.5	2.5	0.0
Trouble with police while drinking	9.5	1.5	2.5
Drinks to forget problems	21.5	9.5	30.0
Ever sought professional help for alcohol problems	4.0	0.0	4.0
Score>3 on Alcohol Problems Scale	16.0	3.5	11.5

consumption of 20 units per week (Royal College of Psychiatrists, 1986). One-third of White and Sikh men reported that they got drunk occasionally, while almost 10% reported that they got drunk at least once every week. The Black sample were significantly less likely to report any of these behaviours – none of the Black men reported becoming intoxicated every week. An even larger proportion (nearly 40% of Sikh and over 22% of Black men) felt that their consumption levels were too high, and substantial minorities of Sikhs and Whites had been advised to moderate their drinking by a GP. Relatively few of the Sikh or Black men reported getting into trouble with the police because of drinking. This is surprising given the suspicion that the police are more likely to notice deviant behaviour in minority groups. An alarmingly high proportion of Sikhs reported that they sometimes drank to forget their problems (iatrogenic drinking), a motive that is commonly assumed to be indicative of an unhealthy relationship with alcohol. Very few Black men exceed the threshold on the Alcohol Problems Scale. The highest proportion of men exceeding a score of three was found among White men. This was partly as a result of the much higher proportion of White men endorsing two items on the scale: admitting that they sometimes got into fights because of their drinking and that they sometimes woke the next day not being able to remember what they had done, while drinking, the night before.

The third aim was to assess trends in drinking patterns across generations. The Sikh and Black groups were divided into those born in Britain (second generation) and those born in the Caribbean or India/East Africa. In both cases there were fewer men in the second generation than the first (85:115 for the Black sample; 38:162 for the Sikh sample). For the Black group, which had a relatively low level of involvement with alcohol overall, there were virtually no differences in the drinking patterns between the generations. For the Sikhs, every index showed a more moderate drinking pattern for the second generation than for the first. There were fewer regular drinkers in the second generation (29 *v.* 48%), those who were regular drinkers in the second generation consumed less alcohol on average (20 *v.* 26 units per week) and significantly fewer of the second generation drank more than 20 units per week (21 *v.* 34%).

The relationship between drinking and demographic variables believed to be related to consumption levels was examined for each of the three ethnic groups to ascertain whether demographic differences related to ethnicity might account for the apparent differences in drinking levels. The only variable on which it was possible to attempt a rough matching before inclusion in the samples was age. Age was strongly related to quantities of alcohol consumed in the White sample (see Table 5) but not in either of the other groups. As expected, young

TABLE 5

Average number of units of alcohol consumed in the past week for three ethnic groups, broken down by demographic variables

	White *n*	White Units	Black *n*	Black Units	Sikh *n*	Sikh Units
Total	200	14	200	6	200	12
Age						
<40	120	17	113	7	119	12
40+	80	10	87	5	81	13
Marital status						
Married	110	13	104	5	152	13
Unmarried	90	15	96	7	48	9
Employment status						
Employed	115	15	102	6	139	13
Unemployed	45	11	98	7	61	10
Social class						
Manual	78	15	128	7	84	10
Non-manual	78	14	47	6	78	15
Student, retired, etc.	44	11	25	3	38	12

White men reported drinking more than older White men; there was a small trend in the same direction for Black men, but not for Sikhs. This ties in with the previous observation about generational differences in drinking patterns for Sikhs where the first generation was both older on average, and drank more, than the second generation. Although Black men were the most likely of the three groups to be unmarried, not employed and in manual jobs, none of these factors was strongly enough related to drinking patterns to account for their (relatively and absolutely) low levels of drinking.

Similarly, the higher proportion of Sikh men who were married, compared with White men, could not by itself account for their relatively higher levels of consumption – even though married Sikhs consumed more alcohol than unmarried Sikhs. This was another reflection of the generational differences, as the first-generation (older) Sikh men were more likely to be married than the second generation. In the Black and White groups being married was associated with lower levels of drinking.

The extent to which religious commitment influenced drinking practices was examined by forming a basic index of religiousness based upon frequency of attendance at religious services (Table 6). There was a consistent pattern across ethnic groups of lower levels of drinking among the more frequent religious attenders; however, this pattern was by no means absolute. For example, 29% of Sikhs who attend temple at least once a week were regular (three times a week or more)

TABLE 6
Alcohol consumption and religious observance

	White (n=200)	Black (n=200)	Sikh (n=200)
Church or temple			
n attending once per week or more	19	58	75
Of which, % regular drinkers	21	10	29
Units per week[1]	10	8	23
n attending once a month or more, but less than once per week	14	12	41
Of which, % regular drinkers	34	17	33
Units per week[1]	23	10	23
n attending occasionally, but less than once per month	65	56	73
Of which, % regular drinkers	39	19	50
Units per week[1]	23	18	26
n not attending at all	102	74	11
Of which, % regular drinkers	39	25	30
Units per week[1]	29	20	13

1. For regular drinkers.

drinkers. What was striking, however, was the relatively low proportion of the White sample who were regular Church attenders (9.5%) compared with regular religious observers among the Black (29%) and Sikh (38%) groups.

Discussion

The question of the reliability of self-reported alcohol consumption must be considered. It is generally accepted that self-report tends to produce underestimates of the amount of alcohol consumed (Crawford, 1987) for a mixture of reasons, such as deliberate deception and forgetfulness. Although it would be desirable to establish accurately the absolute levels of drinking among Black, Sikh and White men, it is accepted that this has not been, and cannot be, achieved using a self-report methodology. It is worth noting that the data on levels of consumption for the White sample in this study are similar to the levels reported in the General Household Survey in 1990 (Office of Population Censuses and Surveys, 1992) where 95% of the male respondents were also White, but where an entirely different methodology was used to estimate consumption levels.

The main issue for the present study is whether the relative drinking levels reported by the three groups are reliable indicators of real differences in the levels of alcohol consumption. In the absence of any direct evidence on this, and given the fact that the self-report data were generally consistent with the data for treated prevalence of alcohol-related problems (Cochrane & Bal, 1989), it might be assumed that the memories and truthfulness of the three ethnic groups are similar, and the data do give a reasonable indication of relative drinking patterns, if not of absolute levels of alcohol consumption. There are, however, two aspects of these data which might undermine this assumption and cannot be disregarded. The Black sample reported that a greater proportion of their consumption was accounted for by spirits than either of the other two samples (Table 3). It is generally accepted that the greatest discrepancy between a standard (pub) measure of alcohol and the amount people pour for themselves exists for spirits. Beer is probably taken in similar size single drinks at home as in a pub and wine might be consumed in somewhat more generous measures at home, but the size of a self-poured measure of spirits might be twice or even three times that poured in a public house. Given that a greater proportion of Black drinking was accounted for by spirits, and that each drink was equated with just one unit, it is possible that the amount of alcohol consumed by the Black sample was underestimated. This would not, of course, affect the estimate of the frequency with which alcohol was taken.

There is also the problem of alcohol amnesias. Responses to an item in the Alcohol Problems Scale indicated that 42% of the White sample and 32% of the Sikh sample (but only 5% of the Black sample) sometimes could not remember what they were doing the night before, when they awoke the morning after a drinking session. This must introduce an element of unreliability into a retrospective measure of drinking employed in this study. Whether or not this unreliability takes the form of a systematic bias in the estimate of levels of alcohol consumption is unclear.

Patterns of alcohol use in minority ethnic groups compared with the native White population

The patterns found in the surveys were generally consistent with the treated prevalence data which were the starting point for the study. Men of African–Caribbean origin reported low levels of consumption and relatively few problems associated with alcohol. Black men were only half as likely to report being regular drinkers than White men, and four times as likely not to drink at all. Even among regular drinkers, Black men drank significantly less each week than White men. Given this, and the fact that there were proportionately fewer Black regular drinkers, it is not surprising that the average consumption level of the entire Black sample was less than half that of the White sample. These findings are consistent with research on the drinking patterns of African Americans (Rebach, 1992).

The Sikh group were more likely to be regular drinkers and drank slightly more on average than the White male group, but the differences found in these surveys were not large enough to explain the large over-representation of Sikh men in hospital admissions. There are three potential explanations for this discrepancy. First, by no means all men born in India who have migrated to Britain are Sikhs. It has been estimated that at least 10% of such immigrants come from White British family backgrounds. It is possible that it is the White migrants from India who account for the high rate of alcohol-related admissions in the Indian-born population, but there is no evidence to support this hypothesis. Second, Asian men may show the deleterious effects of alcohol at a lower consumption threshold than White men. It has been suggested that a liver that is already affected by hepatitis or another factor may more readily incur damage from lower doses of alcohol. If it is the case that the men born in India were exposed to more damage/disease of the liver than UK-born White men, then this could explain their greater vulnerability to alcohol-related illnesses. Finally, Asian men may not use alternative sources of help for alcohol problems to the same extent as White men and are, therefore, more likely to be admitted to mental hospitals. When asked about sources of help for alcohol problems that they might recommend to a friend or relative, Asian men were more likely to suggest the family GP and/or hospital (90%) than were White men (77%). They were less likely (70%) to mention voluntary agencies such as Alcoholics Anonymous than White men (85%). The Asian men were more likely to indicate family and friends as potential sources of help than were the White men.

None of these explanations is conclusive, but each appears consistent with the higher than expected rate of alcohol-related hospital admissions found for Indian-born men.

Level of alcohol-related problems in each group

Total in-patient treatment rates in England indicate a 1.4:1 ratio of White to Black patients admitted to hospitals each year for alcohol-related problems. Evidence from this study on the self-reported incidence of alcohol-related problems suggests that the treated prevalence data are, if anything, an underestimate of the differentials in relative levels of alcohol dependency and serious alcohol problems found among Black and White men. White men were more than twice as likely to consume more than 20 units a week (three times more likely to consume in excess of 30 units), were five times as likely to report episodes of drunkenness, and had four times the rate of exceeding the threshold on the Alcohol Problems Scale. Taking the data from this study, previous surveys and treatment data together, the evidence seems to indicate that Black men in England drink substantially lower quantities of alcohol than do White men and, consequently, have a much lower risk of developing alcohol-related problems.

In one sense this is a surprising finding. One reviewer of American data on minority status and drinking concluded that:

> "Macro-level studies have found rates of alcoholism related to factors that create tension in society... e.g. unemployment rates, family dissolution rates, measures of status integration, and ease of entry to the opportunity structure... These stressors are experienced by greater proportions of minority members and are significant stimuli to subsequent drug and alcohol use..." (Rebach, 1992).

To the extent that Black minorities in Britain share the characteristics of disadvantage evident for African Americans, then it might be predicted that they would manifest higher, not lower, rates of alcohol-related problems. Clearly, some other factors are working against the direct link between social stressors and alcohol misuse in the Black community.

Over 25% of Sikh men drank more than 20 units of alcohol in the week before interview, the highest proportion of any ethnic group (Cochrane & Bal, 1990), and more than 10% exceeded the threshold on the Alcohol Problems Scale. Although this figure is somewhat lower than the equivalent figure for White men (16%), it still gives cause for concern. Alcohol problem scores were significantly higher among older than younger Sikh men – the reverse of the White pattern. There appears to be a subgroup of older, first-generation Sikh men who use alcohol regularly and heavily who experience the expected effects of such use. If the more moderate pattern of alcohol consumption reported by second-generation Sikh men persists as they enter middle age, then the phenomenon of a high level of alcohol-related problems among Sikh men will be a transitory one, which will literally die out with the first generation who are not being replaced by fresh immigrants. Obviously, a cross-sectional study such as this cannot determine whether this will, in fact, be the case or whether the younger second-generation men will adopt the same drinking practices as their fathers as they get older.

Alcohol and religious/cultural factors

The data showed a clear, but not perfect, relationship between frequency of religious attendance and level of alcohol consumption. An examination was also made of the rules governing alcohol use in Christianity and Sikhism. The Granth Sahib states:

> "Drink makes one forget God, and renders one liable to punishment in the Other World. The Guru therefore says, 'Do not drink this liquor, if you wish to swim across the ocean of life'",

and, even more explicitly:

> "Never should a Sikh take wine".

Despite these restrictions in the Granth Sahib, alcohol use is very much a part of Sikh culture. In the Punjab men usually drink alcohol communally in the village centre, and do so playing cards: recreation and alcohol use are synonymous. The same trend may have transferred itself with Sikh men in Britain. The evidence from the present study seems to support this point because Sikhs born in India consume more alcohol than Sikhs born elsewhere. It would be true to say, however, that alcohol as a form of social recreation might equally apply to White working-class men. Certainly the findings of the present study show that both White and Sikh men give socialising as the main reason for drinking.

More Sikh men said they drank every day than did White men. One explanation which can be put forward tentatively for this is the way in which alcohol may be viewed as a 'fortifying' drink. Among Sikh factory workers there is a belief that drinks such as beer and lager have fortifying properties which do more than replenish bodily fluids which are lost through sweating. The belief is that alcoholic beverages enable a man to work harder and longer than if he did not take alcoholic drink, a view which arguably also exists among White working-class men, but to a lesser extent.

Christian religious teaching on alcohol is more ambiguous. There are Old Testament warnings about the dangers of alcohol, for example:

> "Look not thou upon the wine when it is red, when it giveth colour in the cup, when it moveth itself aright. At last it biteth like a serpent, and stingeth like an adder" (Proverbs XXXIII, 31).

However, these appear to be health warnings rather than moral injunctions. The New Testament has positive references to alcohol, as in the miracle at Canna where Jesus turned six stone pots of water into wine for the guests at a wedding and St Paul's famous advice to Timothy, "drink no longer water, but use a little wine for thy stomach sake and thine other infirmities". Of course, wine also plays a central role in the Christian ritual of communion.

Despite the references to the use of alcohol (wine) by Christ and his followers contained in the Bible there has been a very strong temperance movement in Christianity. In its contemporary guise this is manifest in the teachings of some Pentecostal/Evangelical churches in Britain. An undated pamphlet published by The Church of God of Prophecy called *Important Bible Truths* contains the following references to alcohol: "The Bible expressly forbids the use of intoxicating beverages. Even slight indulgence is sinful...," and "The Lords' supper consists of unleavened bread, which represents his body and the wine (unfermented grape juice), which represents the blood of Christ shed for our sanctification".

Seventy per cent of the White sample in our study gave their religious affiliation as either Church of England or Roman Catholic (9% Pentecostal, 21% none). Only 27% of Black men said they adhered to the traditional (British) Christian churches, while 51.5% said they belonged to Pentecostal churches (4% Rastafarian, 18% none).

Adherents to Pentecostal churches are influenced by their teachings, as 49% of the Black men who gave this as their religious affiliation were abstainers. This finding could help to explain the relatively large proportion of the Black sample who reported themselves to be total abstainers.

Not only were Black men more likely to be affiliated to churches which proscribe alcohol use, they were also likely to be involved in religious observances more regularly – nearly one-third were weekly church attenders compared to less than 10% of White men. Those who did go to church regularly were less likely to be regular drinkers than occasional or non-attenders. The regular attenders drank much less on average, even when they were regular drinkers. Thus religion, in terms of its particular teachings and the strength of its influence, is a significant predictor of alcohol consumption, and an important explanatory variable in accounting for differences between Black and White drinking habits.

It is commonly assumed by the White majority in Britain that people of African–Caribbean origin use other and illegal drugs in preference to alcohol, especially cannabis. The present study did not gather data on this question and there appears to be no reliable evidence that illegal drug use is more widespread in the Black than the White community. Indeed, a study by the Home Office Research Unit found that, contrary to the popular stereotype, Black people in Britain were less likely to be involved in drug-related crimes than their White counterparts (*The Guardian*, 4 July 1994).

For the time being, at least, the greater involvement in Christian sects which prohibit alcohol use seems the most likely explanation of the substantially lower level of alcohol consumption reported by Black than White respondents.

References

BALAJARAN, R. & YUEN, P. (1986) British smoking and drinking habits: variation by country of birth. *Community Medicine*, **8**, 237–239.

COCHRANE, R. & BAL, S. S. (1989) Mental hospital admission rates of immigrants to England: a comparison of 1971 and 1981. *Social Psychiatry and Psychiatric Epidemiology*, **24**, 2–11.

—— (1990) The drinking habits of Sikh, Hindu, Muslim and white men in the West Midlands: a community survey. *British Journal of Addiction*, **85**, 759–769.

—— & HOWELL, M. (1995) Drinking patterns of Black and White men in the West Midlands. *Social Psychiatry and Psychiatric Epidemiology*, **30**, 139–146.

CRAWFORD, A. (1987) Bias in a survey of drinking habits. *Alcohol and Alcoholism*, **22**, 167–179.

McKEIGUE, P. M. & KARMI, G. (1993) Alcohol consumption and alcohol-related problems in Afro–Caribbeans and South Asians in the United Kingdom. *Alcohol and Alcoholism*, **28**, 1–10.

OFFICE OF POPULATION CENSUSES AND SURVEYS (1992) *General Household Survey, 1992*. London: HMSO.

REBACH, H. (1992) Alcohol and drug use among American minorities. In *Ethnic and Multicultural Drug Abuse* (eds J. E. Trimble, C. S. Bolek & S. J. Niemcryk), pp. 23–57. New York: Haworth Press.

ROOTMAN, I. & MOSER, J. (1984) *Community Responses to Alcohol Related Problems*. Washington, DC: Department of Health and Human Services.

ROYAL COLLEGE OF PSYCHIATRISTS (1986) *Alcohol: Our Favourite Drug*. London: Tavistock.

9 Practice of child psychiatry in multi-ethnic Britain: some issues and solutions

INDIRA VYAS

A culture's view on the rites of passage and the role of young children and adolescents in the family and society are usually well established. Distress experienced by children and adolescents may be identified by the culture but, as discussed in Chapters 3 and 4, seeking help may depend upon a number of factors. Epidemiological and psychological morbidity data in these two groups are often scanty, especially for children and adolescents belonging to ethnic minorities. This chapter looks at some of the general issues concerning the development of child psychiatry as a speciality, epidemiological data (both within the majority population and among ethnic minority groups) and offers some suggestions for the development of services (see Chapter 22).

Current national status of child psychiatry

Child psychiatry, a relatively new speciality, has existed in Britain since the 1920s. Over the past 30 years the speciality has flourished, with a steady growth in the number of sub-specialists, research, further development of existing skills and development of new ways of helping children and families (Hersov, 1986). Child psychiatry services are now well established in most health districts and are well used by the population.

It would be helpful to look at service provision for ethnic minority children and their families and to compare this with the services provided for the ethnic majority of children and their families in Britain, against the backdrop of the current status of the services nationwide. Child psychiatric services operate either from community-based child guidance clinics administered by local authorities or hospital-based out-patient clinics. Services generally provide assessment, management and treatment for school-age children with emotional and behavioural problems, interpersonal and developmental difficulties, formal psychiatric disorders and for those children who have been victims of abuse. It is usual to assess children in a family setting, sometimes with a co-therapist or a consultation team behind a one-way screen. Child psychiatrists offer psychiatric liaison and consultations with social services, schools, educational psychologists and other primary health workers. They also provide an emergency service for young people who present with psychiatric emergencies, for example, self-harm or psychosis.

Over the past two decades there has been an increase in the number of complex cases, such as all forms of child abuse, which require high levels of special skills, not only in terms of assessment, management and treatment, but also from child psychiatrists in court with regard to medico-legal work.

Resource implications

Children make up 20% of the UK's population. A study of consultations with general practitioners (GPs) has shown that one child in four attending a GP has a psychiatric disorder (Garralde & Bailey, 1986), and that behavioural disorder is the third most common cause for consultation with GPs (Campion & Gabriel, 1984). Yet, child mental health services do not usually receive more than 5% of the mental health budget.

Response of distinguished bodies

In the introduction of the Government report *The Health of the Nation* (Balarajan & Raleigh, 1993), Baroness Cumberlege states categorically that: "The Government is determined that people from ethnic communities should share fully in these improvements". However, there is no mention of child mental health.

Action for Sick Children, in its quality review series, does acknow-ledge that mental health services for children and young people need to address the requirements of children from ethnic minorities (Kurtz, 1992). The excellent survey *Health and Lifestyles: Black and Minority Ethnic Groups in England* by the Health Education Authority includes people over the age of 16 years (Rudat, 1994). A similar, child-centred survey would be desirable.

Change in attitude

In the past 20 years there has been a slow change in attitudes from, at one point, questions being raised about equity of service for all children, irrespective of their ethnic origin, to the backlash of ritual cries of political correctness, insisting that only ethnic minority clinicians could provide child psychiatry services to children of ethnic minorities. Fortunately, it seems that, although the pendulum has had to swing to the extremes, it has come to rest in a more balanced position of genuine understanding of the task ahead (see Chapter 10).

Epidemiology

Prevalence rate

Many community-based epidemiological studies have been undertaken which indicate a prevalence rate of emotional and behavioural problems of 7% for pre-school children, rising to 20% in adolescence (Rutter *et al*, 1970, 1975; Rutter, 1989).

In a classic study, Rutter *et al* (1975) studied 10-year-old children from London and the Isle of Wight and reported that 40% of children with deviant scores on the teacher's questionnaire were found to have definite psychiatric disorders, and that this was more likely with the London sample. A comparison with other schools in London confirmed high rates across London. In the same series Berger *et al* (1975) reported a specific reading retardation in 10% – a figure three times higher than in the Isle of Wight. Rutter *et al* (1975) argued that family discord, parental deviance, social disadvantage and certain school characteristics were key factors in the results. Social disadvantage and inner-city residence are likely to play an important role with children from ethnic minorities.

Special risk factors

(a) Children living in inner-city areas are likely to have twice the prevalence rate of psychiatric disorders (Rutter *et al*, 1975).

(b) Higher rates of disturbance are found in children whose parents have experienced family breakdown. For example, girls under the age of 16 who have become part of a stepfamily are twice as likely to become teenage mothers and three times more likely to leave home before their 18th birthday (Department of Health, 1993). The scale of the problem becomes evident when we realise that in Britain one in four adolescents have experienced parental marital breakdown by the age of 16 years. According to *Social Trends* (Church, 1995), in 1992 the UK had the highest divorce rate in the European Community.

(c) Children whose parents suffer from mental illness, especially those whose mothers suffer from depression, are at increased risk of behavioural problems.

(d) Children with clinical illness and with disability are three times more likely to have behavioural problems (Berger *et al*, 1975)

Epidemiological studies in ethnic minorities

Black children

The available literature (Rutter *et al*, 1974; Earls & Richman, 1980, 1986) suggests that the prevalence of behavioural problems is the same as in the indigenous White community, with a variation in diagnostic type and a difference in gender ratio. However, in West Indian families there was more overcrowding, poor housing and more separation of West Indian children from their mothers, partly due to their history of immigration.

Goodman & Richards (1995) compared second-generation African–Caribbean children with White children and found that they had lower levels of emotional disorders, but psychotic and autistic disorders were proportionally more common.

Asian children

Research in this area is limited and produces conflicting evidence. Early studies (Kallarchal & Herbert, 1976) suggested that Asian children had better mental health, but a more recent study by Newth & Corbett (1993) found similar prevalence of emotional and behavioural problems in Asian and White English children. Hackett's work (see Chapter 10) suggests that Asian (Gujarati) families were less likely to have problems related to divorce. They were also less likely to report fears which were actually higher in the Asian group, thereby suggesting that parents did not feel concerned (Hackett & Hackett, 1993).

Other important factors

There is under-representation of Asian children in child psychiatric services (Stern *et al*, 1990), although there is over-representation of Black children in the care system and residential institutions. This may partly be due to under-recruitment of Black foster-families, although this problem is actively being addressed by most local authorities since The Children Act 1989. Black children are over-represented in the group of children who have been excluded from schools (Bourne *et al*, 1994). To complicate the situation further, long-term unemployment in Britain is highest for Black people at 15.8% compared with the White group which is 4% (Church, 1995). Young Black men are more likely to have negative experiences with the police. They are also more likely to receive custodial sentences. Thus, a multitude of factors are involved in the mental and social health needs of Black children and adolescents. The mental health needs of refugee children who have recently arrived from either war-torn zones or from areas of natural disasters like Ethiopia, Somalia and the former Eastern block remain largely unmet.

Under-representation of Asian children

There may be a lack of knowledge within the Asian community of the availability of child psychiatric services, as many Asian families come from countries where such services are either not readily available or are rudimentary (as has previously been noted in studies of Asian adults). Parents may misinterpret their children's symptoms as physical ill-health or laziness. They may consult their GP about these symptoms, however the GP may make selective referrals (see Chapters 3 and 4).

Like some parents from the indigenous population, Asian parents may be worried about labelling their children as 'mad' or may be reluctant to take their private problems outside of the home. Hackett (see Chapter 10) suggests that parents may experience services as being culturally insensitive or irrelevant to their needs. Like adult patients, parents may seek help from alternative health practitioners. There may also be a genuinely low prevalence rate of disorder in Asian children.

Treatment modalities

Child psychiatry essentially uses a range of talking therapies. The understanding of the culture, nuances in emotional expression, language and family functioning are important, not only to avoid stereotyping, but also to be able to engage and help the family. Services need to develop relevant assessment models, strategies and skills, for which the knowledge of different child-rearing practices, especially in the areas of child abuse and adolescent overdoses, are essential. Assessments need to take into account the differing definition of 'family' and the impact of not only the extended family but also the ancestral family, and the differing gender roles and sibling hierarchies (Vyas, 1991). The migration history of families may explain generational and cultural gaps between parents and their children (see Chapter 10).

Tasks ahead

Department of Health

The Department of Health has expressed great sentiments which need to be strengthened by deeds. These can be assisted by the following.

(a) Ethnic monitoring of all referrals to child psychiatric services (as Bahl has suggested in Chapter 2).
(b) A directive banning the use of children as interpreters for their parents.
(c) A requirement for health districts to provide an appropriate interpreting service when necessary.
(d) Increasing the awareness among parents from ethnic minorities of psychological factors conducive to the emotional well-being of children. A highly successful precedent exists because the Department of Health took steps to educate ethnic minority parents regarding causation of rickets in children and the dangers of applying kohl.
(e) Educating women regarding the prevention of child abuse and raising awareness of child sexual abuse to explode the myth that 'child sexual abuse does not occur in Eastern cultures'. A small local experiment was highly successful.

Commissioners and providers

It is important that health commissioners make adequate provision to provide a comprehensive child mental health service for their districts. They need to ensure: that families from ethnic minorities are aware of the services; that the services are culturally sensitive, relevant and equitable; and that adequate interpreting services are provided.

Training institutions

Bodies like the Royal College of Psychiatrists, the Institute of Family Therapy and the Association of Child Psychotherapists have, to some extent, taken some steps towards including a transcultural dimension to their training, but these need to be extended. It is also important to encourage enrolment of people from ethnic minority groups into training of child psychotherapists.

Employers

Despite the enormous strain on child psychiatric services throughout the country, clinicians continue to aim to provide a culturally appropriate service to its population. The relevant skills may still need to be developed. The trusts which serve populations from ethnic minorities need to facilitate the acquisition of these skills by clinicians.

References

BALARAJAN, R. & RALEIGH, S. V. (1993) *Health of the Nation; Ethnicity and Health. A Guide for the NHS.* London: Department of Health.

BERGER, M., YULE, W. & RUTTER, M. (1975) Attainment and adjustment in two geographical areas: II. Prevalence of specific reading retardation. *British Journal of Psychiatry,* **126**, 510–519.

BOURNE, J., BRIDGES, L. & CHRIS, S. (1994) *Outcast England: How Schools Exclude Black Children.* Nottingham: Russell Press.

CAMPION, P. & GABRIEL, J. (1984) Child consultation patterns in general practice. *British Medical Journal,* **288**, 1426–1428.

CHURCH, J. (ed.)(1995) *Social Trends.* London: HMSO.

DEPARTMENT OF HEALTH (1993) *On the State of Public Health. The Annual Report of the Chief Medical Officer for the Year 1993,* pp. 74–112. London: HMSO.

EARLS, F. & RICHMAN, M. (1980) Behavioural problems in pre-school children of West Indian-born parents; a re-examination of family and social factors. *Journal of Child Psychology and Psychiatry and Allied Disciplines,* **21**, 107–117.

—— & —— (1986) The prevalence of behaviour problems in three year old children of West Indian parents. *Journal of Child Psychology and Psychiatry and Allied Disciplines,* **21**, 99–106.

GARRALDE, M. & BAILEY, D. (1986) Children with psychiatric disorder in primary care. *Journal of Child Psychology and Psychiatry and Allied Disciplines,* **27**, 611–624.

GOODMAN, R. & RICHARDS, H. (1995) Child and adolescent psychiatric presentation of second-generation Afro-Caribbeans in Britain. *British Journal of Psychiatry,* **167**, 362–369.

HACKETT, L., HACKETT, R., & TAYLOR, D. C. (1991) Psychological disturbance and its association in the children of the Gujarati community. *Journal of Child Psychology and Psychiatry,* **32**, 851–856.

—— & HACKETT, R. (1993) Parental ideas of normal and deviant child behaviour. A comparison of two ethnic groups. *British Journal of Psychiatry,* **162**, 353–357.

HERSOV, L. (1986) Child psychiatry in Britain – the last 30 years. *Journal of Child Psychology and Psychiatry and Allied Disciplines,* **27**, 781–801.

KALLARCHAL, A. M. & HERBERT, M. (1976) The happiness of Indian immigrant children. *New Society,* **4**, 22–24.

KURTZ, Z. (1992) *With Health in Mind: Mental Health Care for Children and Young People.* London: Action for Sick Children & S. W. Thames Regional Health Authority.

NEWTH, S. J. & CORBETT, J. (1993) Behavioural and emotional problems in three year old children of Asian parentage, **34**, 333–352.

RUDAT, K. (1994) *Health and Lifestyles: Black and Minority Ethnic Groups in England.* Health Education Authority. Exeter: Wheatstones.

RUTTER, M. (1989) Isle of Wight revisited: twenty-five years of child psychiatric epidemiology. *Journal of the American Academy of Child and Adolescent Psychiatry*, **28**, 633–653.

——, TIZARD, J. & WHITMORE, K. (1970) *Education, Health and Behaviour*. London: Longman.

——, YULE, W., BERGER, M., *et al* (1974) Children of West Indian immigrants – I. Rates of behavioural deviance and psychiatric disorder. *Journal of Child Psychology and Psychiatry and Allied Disciplines*, **15**, 241–262.

——, YULE, B., QUINTAN, B., *et al* (1975) Attainment and adjustment in two geographical areas: III. Some factors accounting for area differences. *British Journal of Psychiatry*, **126**, 520–533.

STERN, G., COTTRELL, D. & HOLMES, J. (1990) Patterns of attendance of child psychiatry out-patients with special reference to Asian families. *British Journal of Psychiatry*, **156**, 384–387.

VYAS, I. (1991) Emotional problems in Asian children – a practical approach. *Newsletter of the Association for Child Psychology and Psychiatry*, **13**, 10–14.

10 Gujarati children in Manchester

RICHARD HACKETT

Psychiatric disorders in children differ from those elsewhere in medicine. While major disorders in adult psychiatry are increasingly seen in physical terms, the disorders that child psychiatrists most commonly diagnose consist of behaviour and emotion that is abnormal in severity, rather than kind, and is rarely accompanied by physical signs of brain disease. Diagnostic labels used by child psychiatrists, such as conduct and emotional disorder, do not, by themselves, usually predict a treatment that will help; this comes from examining the factors that have contributed in each particular case.

Child psychiatrists have always acknowledged the variety of influences that combine to produce behaviours and emotions in children. Some of these factors are particular to the child such as temperament or the effect of injuries to his or her brain (fortunately a rare and sporadic event in Western countries). However, many of the factors that affect children are shared, either within their families, or in a wider social domain such as school, neighbourhood or, in the case of many immigrant groups, community. The very idea of belonging to a community is alien to most White people living in mainstream British life. As discussed in Chapter 1, for an immigrant, belonging to a community can be central to their identity, either because their family comes from a part of the world where society is organised on communal lines, or because the sense of belonging to a distinct community has been thrust upon them by virtue of skin colour and immigration from another country.

Belonging to a minority community can give its members mutual support, as well as a sense of being separate and distinct, but it may also lead to a feeling of vulnerability or persecution. For immigrants of south Asian origin, these communal structures have been imported, directly or indirectly, from the mosaic that is society on the Indian subcontinent. For these people community has meant distinctions of language, details of religious practice and of occupation and ultimately their communities are defined by endogamous rules of marriage.

Though these communities can be defined in a number of ways, it is common for them to have shared attitudes and practices that are transmitted across generations, which in effect constitute part of their culture. They can affect almost any domain of life but are not static, especially in those who have migrated. Some practices are conspicuous (and apparently superficial), such as dress; others are less obvious, such as the way children are brought up. These attitudes and practices constitute an enormous area of shared experience for the members of these communities. If it is true that experiences early in life have profound effects, then culturally determined child-rearing practices may shape not just individuals but entire communities of children and even determine their susceptibility to psychiatric disorder (see Chapter 9).

Parents face many practical tasks that are universal: all children have to be fed, to sleep, to be clothed and bathed. Young children invariably do things their parents do not want them to do and the parent then faces the task of changing the child's behaviour. Though parents may feel as if they are responding to the daily exigencies of life, the way in which they respond will be affected by their own upbringing and how their own parents coped.

Anyone who has interviewed large numbers of parents quickly discovers that parents also have an idea of a 'right' way to bring up their children, even if they sometimes fall short of this ideal. This probably comes from many sources including the media, friends and advice from professionals. Again, it is likely that many of these values come from their parents during their own upbringing and in this sense the ideas are cultural.

The practical tasks of child-rearing can also be vehicles for the parents' values, and will affect how the children approach the task when it is their turn. In this way child-rearing can transmit communal values.

Though communities may be responsible for broad shifts in child-rearing practices and parental attitude, there will always be differences in parenting style from one family to another. To separate the two, representative samples of adequate size have to be examined.

We have studied Manchester's Gujarati community (Hackett *et al*, 1991; Hackett & Hackett, 1993, 1994) and attempted to explore the relationship between child-rearing practices, parents' ideas of normal and abnormal behaviour and psychiatric disorders in children. The original impetus for the studies was the observation that the children of immigrants of south Asian origin were under-represented in child psychiatry clinics in Manchester. In retrospect, this observation was probably correct only for certain Asian communities in some parts of Manchester.

Manchester's Gujarati community

During the latter part of the 19th century many Indians, especially from Gujarati-speaking areas, were encouraged to go to east Africa, usually as indentured labour. Ultimately, their conspicuous successes brought the Indian immigrants problems, particularly in Uganda, from which they were expelled in the 1970s. Many arrived in Britain and settled in communities in large cities and towns, including Oldham and Ashton-under-Lyne in east Manchester. This particular community now consists of approximately 800 families but it is not entirely homogeneous, consisting of three largely endogamous groupings united by Hinduism and the Gujarati language. These families have retained strong links with India and have frequently brought over marriage partners from India. By the late 1980s a generation of their children had been born in Britain, and they were the subjects of our studies. Though attending state schools, many of these children still go to Gujarati language classes in the evenings. Temples have been established, sometimes in converted terrace houses, and the community still tends to cluster in a few residential areas served by Gujarati-oriented provision shops.

The study

Constraints of time and manpower limited the studies to a sample of 100 Gujarati families who had children aged between four and seven years. We eventually gathered our sample through schools that had a high intake of children from the Gujarati community. The headteachers generally preferred to approach the parents themselves, aided by a leaflet in Gujarati explaining the intentions of the study. Before this we had put up notices in temples and Gujarati shops.

The attitude of the schools and particularly the Gujarati people themselves was very helpful. Far from viewing our intrusion with suspicion they cooperated enthusiastically. The White sample was recruited from the same schools using a standard letter. Though active refusals were very rare, the failure of many parents to respond to the invitation probably biased this sample.

The information was gathered using a questionnaire administered to the Gujarati parents by an Indian psychiatrist with a facility in Hindi. I administered the questionnaire to the White control group parents. The interview elicited information about child-rearing practices in a number of domains and these items owed much to Newson's major study of four-year-olds (Newson & Newson, 1968). The areas covered included: the inculcation of physical and social independence, tolerance of disruptive play and temper tantrums, attitudes to violence and lying, disciplinary practices, toilet-training, feeding, sleeping arrangements, attitudes to ownership and possessions, habits and the expectation of obedience. In addition Rutter's Behaviour Scale for Completion by Parents (Rutter *et al*, 1970) was administered as a measure of psychological disturbance. Help was sought from a member of the Gujarati community for the translation of the questionnaire before the interviews began.

A number of strategies were employed in the questionnaire items. Some of the information was factual, such as the age at which toilet-training was started or the time at which the children went to bed, or whether they took a comfort object with them. In addition, parents were frequently asked whether they were satisfied with their child's behaviour or performance in the various domains. We made the assumption that an expectation of early achievement or expressions of dissatisfaction with performance (where the actual performance between children did not significantly differ) indicated more stringent attitudes and the attachment of greater importance by parents to these behaviours. Another way in which the practices and attitudes of parents were assessed was by the use of vignettes which described situations familiar to any parent. Thus, one of the items aimed at assessing the extent to which parents either tolerated or discouraged aggression consisted of asking parents how they would want their child to react if the child was hit for no apparent reason by another child while in the school playground. Obedience to parental authority was assessed by asking parents how they responded when they wanted their child to tidy up some toys but the child wanted to continue watching television. Sometimes parents were simply asked how strongly they felt about particular areas of child behaviour. For others, such as temper tantrums, they were asked whether they were happy to let children grow out of the behaviour or whether they actively suppressed the behaviour.

There were very few problems of translation, which probably reflects the universal nature of the issues we were investigating. However, the problems of equivalence we did come across were informative. We had difficulty finding a Gujarati phrase that conveyed the same connotation of wilfulness contained in the phrase 'temper tantrum'. It appeared that there were fundamental differences in the way parents viewed this particular behaviour. White parents saw it as essentially a confrontation, whereas the phrase used by Gujarati parents tended to emphasise the distress of the child. Indeed, many Gujarati parents expressed amazement at the confrontations they witnessed in supermarkets between White children demanding a toy and their parents refusing. Problems in finding lexical equivalence contain valuable pointers to cultural differences (see Chapter 5).

Results

The social class of the two samples differed, with skilled and semi-skilled fathers being over-represented among the Gujarati sample; professional and managerial parental occupations were over-represented among the White sample. We did not ascertain whether migration had forced the Gujarati parents to take lower status jobs when they arrived in Britain. If this were so, their Office of Population Censuses and Surveys social class could be misleading. Though the age at which mothers finished full-time education was 16 years in both groups, the spread was greater among the Gujarati sample including two mothers who had never attended school. One-parent families were more common in the White than the Gujarati sample. Gujarati families were more likely to have grandparents or aunts and uncles living with them. The size of sibships was significantly greater among the Gujarati families.

The vignette concerning physical aggression elicited different responses from the two groups of parents. Far more of the Gujarati parents insisted that their child tell a teacher, rather than hit the child back, whereas the majority of White parents preferred their child to retaliate. Most of the Gujarati parents said they would disapprove were their child to hit back, whereas most of the White parents were happy for their child to do so. One Gujarati parent said that if the assailant were White, her son should retaliate, but if he or she was Asian he should not! In another vignette parents were asked how they would want their child to respond if another child snatched a toy from him or her while they were playing outside. The findings precisely reflected those in the previous vignette; far more of the White parents expected their child to violently repossess the toy, whereas most of the Gujarati children were expected to come into the house and tell their parents or persuade the other child to return the toy.

Gujarati parents exerted more pressure on their children to share and expected their child to acquiesce to the disposal of their property, signalling less respect for the individual property rights of children. However, White parents were more likely to actually give toys or clothes away (for instance, to jumble sales) but usually used subterfuge when doing so.

The Gujarati parents had higher expectations of obedience and were less tolerant of disruptive play in the home such as using furniture for make-believe, making a mess with earth, water or paint or making a lot of noise. Temper tantrums were less common among the Gujarati children and their parents were much less tolerant of them, most feeling that children should have grown out of them by the age of the child under study. Many of them felt that such behaviour had to be actively suppressed, while more of the White parents felt that their children would grow out of it. When this behaviour arose, Gujarati parents relied on reprimand or explanation whereas the White parents preferred to ignore, shame or tease the child. Gujarati parents were more likely to reward their children for good behaviour, and threaten them with an authority figure or threaten to send the child away (usually to an aunt in London) when other misbehaviour occurred. They were also more likely to tell the child that they did not love them, a strategy that elicited strong disapproval from the White parents whose preferred method of discipline was sending the child to bed. Though significantly more White than Gujarati parents felt that smacking was necessary, the samples did not differ in the frequency with which they admitted to using smacking. Surprisingly, the attitude towards lying was less lenient among White parents than Gujarati parents.

Expectations of physical independence in terms of dressing, using a toilet independently and other self-care tasks did not differ. The Gujarati parents, however, appeared to expect their children to be able to concentrate for longer.

The Gujarati parents had significantly severer attitudes to toilet-training as they preferred to start it at a mean age of 10 months compared with 17 months among the White parents. Their attitude to bedwetting was also more condemnatory and, perhaps unsurprisingly, their children did it less often.

Fear of spiders, the dark, dogs and other commonly encountered objects was far more common among Gujarati children, but their parents were no more concerned by their children having extensive fears than were White parents. In fact, Gujarati parents tolerated more fears than did their White counterparts.

Sleeping arrangements were markedly different between the two samples. Gujarati children went to bed later, and if they did not seem tired, their parents were much less likely to insist that they still go to bed. On both counts the White parents enforced an early and strict bedtime. More White children took a comfort object, such as a teddy bear, to bed with them or insisted on a bedtime ritual. Once in bed, fewer of them were allowed back downstairs. The Gujarati children were much more likely to share the bed, and to a later age. White children usually slept in a cot in their parents room that was removed on average at the age of 8 months. Gujarati children, on the other hand, usually slept in their parent's bed until they had reached a mean age of 3 years 3 months.

Few clear trends emerged when feeding practices were compared. Gujarati parents weaned their children later than Whites, but breast-fed less.

Using a standard cut-off on the Rutter Scale, 21% of White children were disturbed compared with just 5% of the Gujarati children, a significant difference. In both groups physical independence was associated with the absence of psychological disturbance. Among the White children psychological disturbance was associated with separation from parents during early childhood, whereas among the Gujarati children it was not.

Discussion

Critique of the method

Many methodological criticisms can be made of this study, such as its small size and the unrepresentativeness of the samples, especially the White control families, among whom the most socially integrated were likely to have volunteered.

Criticisms can also be made of the questions and instruments used to measure behaviour and attitudes. Rutter's scales have been widely used among White children, but use of them among non-indigenous communities assumes that these children show distress in exactly the same way as White children. This assumption has already been questioned in a study of adults belonging to other immigrant communities. Rack (1984) described 'reactive excitation' among African–Caribbean people and somatisation among Pakistani immigrants (Rack, 1982); in both cases he suggested that these were culture-specific idioms of distress. As highlighted in Chapters 4 and 5, Kleinman (1977, 1987) argued that cases in a different culture should only be counted after defining them in accordance with conceptions of deviance specific to that culture, otherwise there would be a risk of labelling groups of children as abnormal who would not be viewed as such by members of their own community. Indeed, Kleinman argued that the very categories used by Western psychiatrists were alien and inappropriate. Much has been made of this by psychiatrists with an anthropological orientation. For them, the imposition of Western concepts of psychiatric disorder represents the cardinal sin of 'category fallacy' (Kleinman, 1987). This position of rigid cultural relativism assumes that the edifice of Western psychiatry is of no utility outside its own culture, but it risks being undermined by the burgeoning research into the biological mechanisms that underlie much major psychiatric disorder in adults (see Chapter 6), and may yet do the same for children. To use an example from adult psychiatry, if an individual in a remote part of Africa hears voices that distress him or her, regardless of whether his or her experience is viewed as being due to possession by evil spirits or a brain disorder, consumption of a suitable neuroleptic drug in an adequate dose is likely to make him or her feel better. However, cultural factors impinge on even the most organic disease model; this individual's view of his or her disease would very likely determine whether he or she takes the small white objects that he or she has been instructed to swallow (the distinction between disease and illness; see Chapter 4).

Even among Whites in Britain, the idea that misbehaviour and unhappiness in children can be viewed as disorders (of conduct and emotion) is frequently alien, so category fallacies can be committed by White psychiatrists on White patients.

Child-rearing

As stated before, child-rearing has some universal themes and there are some behaviours that would worry parents anywhere in the world. Within the behaviours that we enquired about, it seems that rather than completely different behaviours being of concern to the two communities, parents differed in the threshold at which they considered a particular behaviour abnormal or unacceptable. Thus, we found that the Gujarati parents were far less tolerant of physical aggression, temper tantrums, disobedience and disruptive play in the home. They also had higher expectations with regard to toilet-training. In practical terms, behaviour that would be viewed as healthy self-assertion by the parents of a White child might be considered worryingly aggressive by a Gujarati parent were their child to act in the same way. The more stringent attitude of Gujarati parents towards these behaviours would lead to a lower threshold at which they would consider them to be abnormal. One implication of this for the use of instruments that measure behaviour is that some items should be more heavily weighted when Gujarati families are being observed. Conversely, the White parents were less tolerant of lying and fears in their children, so, in a comparative study such as ours, these two behaviours should be given more weight as evidence of psychological disturbance when they are observed in White British children.

Cultural differences in ideas of normal and deviant behaviour present the children of immigrant communities with conflicts on an almost daily basis. Though we did not study older children, the potential conflicts for teenagers are still greater. Behaviour that would be normal in a 15-year-old White girl would cause outrage if displayed by her Gujarati counterpart looking towards an arranged marriage.

Implications for clinical practice

If a Gujarati child is referred to a clinic because the parents feel the child is excessively violent, should the clinician consider the child's behaviour from the point of view of their community, in which case efforts might be directed at altering the child's behaviour, or should the clinician assess the child's behaviour in the light of White British values, which are far more tolerant towards aggression, in which case the psychiatrist should attempt to alter the parents' expectations.

The central finding of the study, that Gujarati children enjoy greater psychological well-being than their White British counterparts, offers an explanation for their under-representation in child psychiatry clinics. However, the possibility that child psychiatric services may not be fully utilised for other reasons by minority ethnic groups should be considered. Other studies that have looked at south Asian immigrant communities (Kallarackal & Herbert, 1976) also showed lower indices of psychological disturbance in their south Asian samples, though they treated these samples as homogeneous groupings; this is a methodological weakness of considerable importance. In Rutter *et al*'s (1974) study of African–Caribbean children in London, teachers reported high rates of psychological disturbance but parents did not. Perhaps the children exhibited different behaviour at school, or perhaps African–Caribbean parents and White British teachers view the same behaviour differently. We do not know which of these possibilities is true.

The simplistic notion that having a non-White skin automatically puts the individual at greater risk of psychiatric disorder may be true in adults (see Chapter 5), but is not sustained by this study of Gujarati children. Being a population-based study, under-reporting of disorders is unlikely to explain their relative psychological well-being. Cochrane (1979) suggested that either the process of Asian migration selected psychologically robust individuals and these characteristics were passed on to their children, or their family structures helped to prevent psychological disturbance.

Family structure

Our findings cannot shed light on the psychological characteristics before migration, but we certainly did find evidence of more favourable family structures. Ten per cent of the White children in our study had only one parent living with them compared with 3% of the Gujarati children. In addition, the Gujarati one-parent families were much more likely to have close contact with second-degree relatives such as grandparents or aunts and uncles, who would presumably contribute to the parenting of the child, both practically and in terms of attachment. Interestingly, separation from parents had different consequences for the child. This is probably due to the differing reasons for separation in the two communities. In the White group separation is likely to represent major family dislocations such as divorce, whereas among the Gujarati group   the 'farming-out' of children is a common and benign practice.

Further reasons why the Gujarati children fared better psychologically may be found when child-rearing practices are examined in more detail. As previously mentioned, these are, at one level of description, the response of parents to the universal needs of children. But beyond this, communal differences in how these tasks are executed constitute vehicles for implanting values, and it is these values that may protect children psychologically or expose them. The underlying meanings of these practices have to be examined.

Sleep patterns

Our study demonstrated profound community-wide differences in where, with whom and how children go to sleep. The thread that runs through Gujarati practices in this area was one of nurture and child-centredness. Though we treated them as a minority worthy of study, in this area it is the Gujarati families that conform to wider human (and mammalian) norms in that solitary sleeping is largely limited to Europeans and North Americans. To suggest that this is purely an artefact of living space, and therefore wealth, is refuted by studies showing the extent of co-sleeping in wealthy cultures such as the Japanese (Caudhill & Plath, 1966). Indeed there are many strands of evidence suggesting that Gujarati practices of co-sleeping are more consonant with biological needs (Harlow & Harlow, 1962; Lozoff & Brittenham, 1979; Hunziker & Barr, 1986). But beyond this evidence that close proximity between mother and infant is essential for early attachment and subsequent social development is the social message of co-sleeping: that of communality. This is in stark contrast to the early and severe insistence on individuality that comprises White sleeping practices – inflexible bedtimes combined with solitary sleeping. Interestingly, it has been suggested before (Hong, 1978) that the use of comfort objects by young children assists them to differentiate between self and non-self. The widespread use of them by the White sample, but their near-absence among the Gujaratis, provides further support for the contention that the White British families attach greater importance to individuality compared with the Gujarati community.

Further evidence that communality is an important value among the Gujarati community comes from the emphasis on sharing. The interesting question is whether this communal ethos plays a part in maintaining the psychological well-being of children. One can speculate that it provides a sense of security as well as identification with a group among whom shame would have a strongly controlling effect on misbehaviour.

Social values

The social values that are conveyed by stricter toilet-training among the Gujarati families are worth considering. This represents one of the first opportunities for conflict between parents and their child. The infant's urge is to defaecate where and when it pleases, and that of the parent is to inculcate defaecation at prescribed times and places. The underlying issue and message is one of control, particularly self-control, and this study indicates that it is valued more among the Gujarati than the White community. Further evidence for greater importance being attached to control is the stricter attitude of the Gujarati parents to temper tantrums and aggression. This ethos of constraint permeates the child-rearing practices of the community we studied. Weisz *et al* (1987) also tried to relate social values to the predominant type of psychiatric disorder in children. They compared a community in Thailand, where constraint was strongly encouraged among the young, with the USA where a more liberal atmosphere prevailed. They found that in Thailand children were prone to disorders of over-control, by which they meant emotional disorders, whereas in the USA children were more likely to have disorders of under-control, which equated with conduct disorder. From this it can readily be seen why Gujarati children should be less prone to disorders of under-control, the most common type of disorder in White children.

Anthropologists have wondered why communities have particular value systems that underpin their child-rearing practices. A common explanation is that they are economically adaptive; indeed it has been asserted that the economic and social environment directly shape child-rearing practices, and that a structure of values subsequently arises to justify them (Minturn & Lambert, 1964). The Gujarati community in Manchester remains close-knit and interdependent, socially and economically. It is easy to see why behaviours that promote this would be reinforced during childhood, and those that are detrimental to the integrity of the community will be suppressed. Thus, value is attached to obedience and self-restraint; to do otherwise would threaten the social order. For the same reason the balance between communality and individuality is tilted firmly in favour of the former, and child-rearing practices specifically promote this. Perhaps this is one aspect of the culture of some of the south Asian enclave communities that indigenous Whites are least able to comprehend: that there is an alternative to the Western sense of 'self' based on individuality.

The psychological well-being of these Gujarati children can be seen as a result of their communal values. The relatively secure families in which these children grow up enable their stringent expectations of behaviour to be implemented effectively.

Conclusions

Remarkably little is known about psychiatric disorder in the children of immigrants. The body of knowledge that exists is so patchy that our attempt to understand what is happening to the children of these communities is like trying to guess what a large and complicated jigsaw puzzle will show when only three pieces are in place. The problem is made all the greater because the picture is constantly changing as each community seeks an equilibrium between assimilation and identification. Those engaged in the academic study of these communities should have no illusions that the publication of papers in learned journals will have much influence on the outcome of Britain's immigrant communities' social and economic struggles. However, research findings are needed to leaven the debate and counterbalance the posturing of so many of its participants.

References

CAUDHILL, W. & PLATH, D. W. (1966) Who sleeps by whom? Parent–child involvement in urban Japanese families. *Psychiatry*, **29**, 344–353.

COCHRANE, R. (1979) Psychological and behavioural disturbance in West Indians, Indians and Pakistanis in Britain: a comparison of rates among children and adults. *British Journal of Psychiatry*, **134**, 201–210.

HACKETT, L., HACKETT, R. & TAYLOR, D. C. (1991) Psychological disturbance and its associations in the children of the Gujarati community. *Journal of Child Psychology and Psychiatry and Allied Disciplines*, **32**, 851–856.

—— & —— (1993) Parental ideas of normal and deviant child behaviour. A comparison of two ethnic groups. *British Journal of Psychiatry*, **162**, 353–357.

—— & —— (1994) Child-rearing practices and psychiatric disorder in Gujarati and British children. *British Journal of Social Work*, **24**, 191–202.

HARLOW, H. F. & HARLOW, M. K. (1962) Social deprivation in monkeys. *Scientific American*, **207**, 136.

HONG, K. (1978) The transitional phenomena: a theoretical integration. *Psychoanalytic Study of the Child*, **33**, 47–79.

HUNZIKER, V. A. & BARR, R. G. (1986) Increased carrying reduces infant crying: a randomised controlled trial. *Pediatrics*, **77**, 641–648.

KALLARACKAL, A. M. & HERBERT, M. (1976) The happiness of Indian immigrant children. *New Society*, 26 February, 422–424.

KLEINMAN, A. (1977) Depression, somatisation and the new 'cross-cultural psychiatry'. *Social Science and Medicine*, **11**, 3–10.

—— (1987) Anthropology and psychiatry: the role of culture in cross-cultural research on illness. *British Journal of Psychiatry*, **151**, 447–454.

LOZOFF, B. & BRITTENHAM, G. (1979) Infant care: cache or carry. *Journal of Pediatrics*, **95**, 478–483.

MINTURN, L. & LAMBERT, M. M. (1964) *Mothers of Six Cultures: Antecedents of Child-Rearing*. New York: John Wiley and Sons.

NEWSON, J. & NEWSON, E. (1968) *Four-Years-Old in an Urban Community*. London: Allen & Unwin.

RACK, P. (1982) *Race, Culture and Mental Disorder.* London: Tavistock.
—— (1984) Psychiatric disorders in immigrants. *Readings in Psychiatry,* **3**, 53–57.
RUTTER, M., TIZARD, J. & WHITMORE, K. (1970) *Education, Health and Behaviour.* London: Longman.
——, YULE, W., BERGER, M., *et al* (1974) Children of West Indian immigrants – I. Rates of behavioural deviance and psychiatric disorder. *Journal of Child Psychology and Psychiatry and Allied Disciplines,* **15**, 241–262.
WEISZ, J. R., SUWANLERT, S., CHAIYASIT, W., *et al* (1987) Epidemiology of behavioural and emotional problems among Thai and American children: parents' reports for ages 6 to 11. *Journal of the American Academy of Child and Adolescent Psychiatry,* **26**, 890–897.

11 Cross-cultural approaches to dementia and depression in older adults

MARCUS RICHARDS and MELANIE ABAS

The detection and management of dementia and depression among ethnic minority elders has received relatively little attention, even though these disorders are associated with considerable disability and suffering. We will attempt to describe the complex clinical issues that surround the detection and management of dementia and depression in a cross-cultural setting. However, the consideration of any construct from different perspectives and in different contexts inevitably leads to questions about the nature of that construct. We will also explore some of the ways in which cross-cultural studies can challenge and enrich our conceptions of dementia and depression.

Dementia

Both DSM–IV (American Psychiatric Association, 1994) and ICD–10 (World Health Organization (WHO), 1992) criteria for dementia require the demonstration of cognitive impairment of sufficient severity to interfere with activities of daily living. Yet most formal tests of cognitive function are culture-dependent and societies vary in the degree to which they place functional responsibilities upon their elders. With regard to cognitive function, DSM–IV criteria for dementia state that:

> "Cultural and educational background should be taken into consideration in the evaluation of an individual's mental capacity. Individuals from certain backgrounds may not be familiar with the information used in certain tests (of cognitive function)".

106

Similarly, DSM–IV criteria for dementia acknowledge the importance of culture in assessing functional capacity:

"The nature and degree of (functional) impairment are variable and often dependent on the particular social setting of the individual".

Similar qualifications are made by ICD–10:

"How such a decline (in intellectual and functional capacity) manifests itself will depend largely on the social and cultural setting in which the patient lives".

It is important to explore these qualifications in more detail.

Cognitive assessment

While cognitive tests used in cross-cultural research should be as culture-fair as possible, at least two kinds of bias can be distinguished. The first is test bias, arising from inappropriate item selection, such as items that translate poorly from one language to another or those that represent objects or entities that are unfamiliar to different cultures(see Chapters 4 and 5 for a discussion).

Minimisation of test bias is not, however, a sufficient process. Different cultures have different patterns of experience which influence performance during cognitive testing. Some of these experiences can be formalised, the most important examples being education and occupation. However, the difficulty of equating cultures for level of education and type of occupation should not be minimised, even among cultures of comparable levels of socio-economic development. Second, there are more subtle cultural influences on test performance which are difficult to eliminate, equate or even quantify. As noted by Serpell (further details available from the author upon request), cultures vary in the readiness with which they will display their intellectual skills to strangers and in their familiarity with the conventions of information elicitation outside the context of practical activities. If the assessment of cognitive function is to be undertaken in a cross-cultural setting, test items should have comparable meaning, familiarity and salience across cultures. Such assessment should also be grounded in a proper understanding of the experience and expectations that different cultures bring to the test situation.

Functional assessment

If the assessment of cognitive function in a cross-cultural setting challenges our capacity to bridge the gap between ability and performance, the assessment of functional capacity in a similar context raises important questions about the ecology and expression of dementia in everyday life. A useful framework to approach these questions is provided by the WHO *International Classification of Impairments, Disabilities, and Handicaps* (WHO, 1980). This document draws a distinction between: (a) impairment, which refers to any loss or abnormality of psychological, physiological or anatomical structure or function; (b) disability, which refers to any restriction or lack of ability (resulting from the impairment) to perform tasks, skills and behaviours considered normal for any particular person; and (c) handicap, which refers to the disadvantage (resulting from an impairment or disability) that limits or prevents the fulfilment of a normal role within the boundaries of demographic and cultural expectations. In the case of dementia, neural degeneration constitutes the impairment, while the consequent loss of ability to perform normal activities of daily living defines the disability. Handicap is a more subtle concept, and addresses the value attached to departure from a functional norm. Whether dementia is experienced as a handicap depends on a labelling process performed by the individual, the individual's peers or the wider group setting. This labelling determines, in part, the practical consequences of impairment and disability, both within an individual's kinship network and in relation to health care professionals.

It is important, therefore, to consider the extent to which different cultures label the symptoms of dementia as pathological or normal for old age. This, in turn, depends on cultural expectations of the elderly. In many industrialised societies, it is common for older people to continue to face challenges routinely met by younger adults, such as domestic maintenance and financial management. In such cultures, an older person who is having difficulty with such activities is typically labelled as functionally impaired and is relatively easy to identify. Yet what of cultures that place few functional responsibilities upon their elders? It could be argued that absence of a tendency to 'pathologise' disability only hinders identification of dementia in its early stages and that dementia will be readily detected once it is sufficiently severe to cause behavioural disturbance. However, mortality associated with dementia is high in such rural communities (Chandra *et al*, 1994). Consequently, the later stage of more symptomatic dementia is not always reached(Chandra *et al*, 1999; Fillenbaum *et al*, 1999).

Another difficulty in the cross-cultural assessment of functional ability is the variable prevalence of co-existing physical impairments, such as sensory impairment and arthritis, that can mask functional disability resulting from cognitive decline. These tend to be more prevalent in developing countries, providing a greater challenge for clinicians in these countries to make accurate differential diagnoses (Chandra *et al*, 1994).

Cross-cultural studies of dementia prevalence

Populations of African origin

Osuntokun *et al* (1992) from the University of Ibadan, Nigeria, have made the abrupt statement that: "no authenticated case of Alzheimer's disease has been reported in an indigenous Black African". This statement is based on door-to-door prevalence studies in the Ibadan region (Osuntokun *et al*, 1987; Ogunniyi *et al*, 1992) of consecutive admissions to the University College Hospital, Ibadan, over a period of 30 years, and one post-mortem series (Osuntokun *et al*, 1990). Reports of a collaborative study to compare prevalence rates of dementia in Black Nigerians from Ibadan and African Americans from Indiana indicate that cases of Alzheimer's disease have now been identified in Nigeria (Hendrie *et al*, 1995). Nevertheless, the prevalence of dementia in Nigeria still appears to be lower than among African Americans. There are several possible reasons for this.

First, diagnostic criteria developed in the USA or Western Europe may not be easily adaptable for developing countries, as discussed above. Second, it may be that selective mortality in Nigerians with dementia is high, thus reducing the likelihood of detecting cases at a single point in time. Incidence studies are necessary to resolve this difficulty. Third, although Osuntokun and colleagues do not address the question of whether the symptoms of dementia in old age are labelled normal or pathological within Nigerian culture, it is possible that cases of dementia were concealed from investigators because of social stigma attached to this syndrome. However, in one prevalence survey (Osuntokun *et al*, 1987) it was claimed that virtually all eligible residents were known to study staff. Fourth, the possibility remains that Black African populations are genuinely at low risk for dementia. In support of this possibility, Osuntokun *et al* (1994) reported significantly lower rates of A4-amyloid deposition in a consecutive series of post-mortem brains of patients without dementia from Ibadan, compared with an equivalent series from Melbourne, Australia. It is not clear whether this putative low risk has an environmental locus or is the result of ethnic differences in biological (e.g. genetic, cardiovascular) disposition, or is an interaction between these two factors.

In contrast, African Americans appear to be at a higher risk of dementia. Indeed, two population-based studies found a higher prevalence of dementia among African Americans than among White Americans. In the first of these, Schoenberg *et al* (1985) screened 8925 residents aged 40 years and older in Copiah County, Mississippi, for severe dementia. Of these, 49.1% were African Americans. The age-adjusted prevalence rate for severe dementia was 817 per 100 000 for White people and 987.2 per 100 000 for African American people.

Heyman *et al* (1991) complied a stratified random sample of 83 African American and 81 White community residents aged 65 years and older from the Piedmont region of North Carolina. A total of 26 residents were found to have dementia, yielding a dementia prevalence of 16% for African American people and 3.05% for White people. The prevalence of both Alzheimer's disease and mixed or multi-infarct dementia was higher in the African American subjects.

Populations of Asian origin

Studies of dementia and cognitive impairment in the Asian continent are of particular interest because the proportion of the population aged 65 years and older is growing rapidly (Siegel & Hoover, 1982). Several studies conducted in China have reported a low prevalence of dementia, ranging from 0.46% to 1.86% (Zhang *et al*, 1990). Li *et al* (1989) surveyed 1331 community residents of Beijing and reported a similar dementia prevalence of 1.82% for subjects aged 65 years and older. Zhang *et al* (1990) argue that differences in population structure, in survey methodology and in the application of diagnostic criteria account for this effect. In their own study of 5055 older community residents of Shanghai, they standardised their application of DSM–III (American Psychiatric Association, 1980) and National Institute for Neurological, Communicable Diseases and Stroke–Alzheimers Disease and Related Disorders Association (NINCDS–ADRDA) dementia criteria (McKhann *et al*, 1984) to current practice in the USA. Using a two-phase survey methodology, a dementia prevalence of 4.6% was reported for subjects aged 65 years and older. This figure is comparable to that for Western European and North American countries (Breteler *et al*, 1992). As well as standardisation of diagnostic procedure, two important differences between this and previous studies in China were the use of a more comprehensive clinical assessment of dementia and the use of a screening cut-point to identify cognitive impairment in Phase I of the survey that was adjusted for level of education.

Populations of European origin

Several comprehensive reviews of the epidemiology of dementia in Western Europe and in predominantly White communities in North America have been published (Henderson, 1986; Jorm, 1990; Breteler *et al*, 1992). It is generally assumed that differences between these communities in educational attainment, familiarity with formal cognitive tests and conceptions of normality regarding cognitive and functional capacity in the elderly are smaller in comparison to the developing countries. In this regard, a meta-analysis found no significant difference in the prevalence of dementia across Finland, Italy, Spain, Sweden and the UK (Hofman *et al*, 1991). It should be noted, however, that Treves *et al* (1986) found a significantly higher prevalence of dementia in Jewish people of European origin than in Jewish people of Asian or African origin.

Risk factors for dementia

One potential gain of cross-cultural prevalence and incidence studies of dementia is the provision of insights into dementia aetiology. As Osuntokun *et al* (1992) point out, the identification of ethnic groups with significantly different prevalence rates of dementia could enhance the search for dementia risk factors. Furthermore, the comparison of communities in different environments and at different stages of economic development, but within the same ethnic group, may enable the delineation of environmental from genetic risk factors. A meta-analysis by the EURODEM Risk Factors Research Group (Van Duijn *et al*, 1991) revealed a number of significant risk factors for Alzheimer's disease. These are a family history of dementia, Parkinson's disease or Down's syndrome, head trauma with loss of consciousness, a history of hypothyroidism and a history of depression. In addition, having ever smoked emerged as a protective factor. Unfortunately, no data are available on cross-cultural comparisons of these risk factors.

In line with recent reports (American Heart Association, 1995; National Heart, Lung and Blood Institute, 1995) Heyman *et al* (1991) found that African American people were more likely than White people to have had a history of strokes, hypertension and diabetes. This raises the question of ethnic differences in risk for vascular-related dementia. Some clues to these differences have come from clinical studies. Still *et al* (1990) compiled a case register of patients in South Carolina diagnosed with dementia since April 1988. They reported that although the proportion of African American people did not exceed one-third of South Carolina's population, African

Americans accounted for 44.3% of all dementia cases. Furthermore, although there was no difference between African American people and White people in the proportion of Alzheimer's and multi-infarct dementia cases, the frequency of alcohol-related dementia was higher among African American people. Autopsy studies report conflicting results. Miller *et al* (1984) found no difference between African American and White people in the neuritic plaque and neuro-fibrilliary tangle count in the temporal regions of 199 consecutive post-mortem brains. De la Monte *et al* (1989) studied 144 histo-logically confirmed cases of dementia among 6000 consecutive post-mortem brains. They reported an equal proportion of African American and White subjects among the dementia cases. African American people, however, had a higher proportion of multi-infarct and alcohol-related dementia. White people had a higher proportion of classical Alzheimer's disease pathology and dementia associated with Parkinson's disease. The difficulties in extrapolating clinical data to the population at large are well known (Richards & Chaudhuri, 1996). For example, in the case of mild Alzheimer's disease, African American people may be less likely than White people to come to the attention of a clinician and will therefore be under-represented in clinical series. De la Monte *et al*'s (1989) finding of a higher proportion of cerebrovascular lesions among African American patients is consistent with population-based studies showing a higher frequency of cardiovascular risk factors in this ethnic group.

A summary observation by Jorm (1990) concerning Asian popu-lations is that vascular dementia is more frequently diagnosed than Alzheimer's disease in Japan, China and Russia. However, Jorm points out that this may reflect regional differences in diagnostic practice rather than differences in the true prevalence of these subtypes of dementia. On the other hand, the incidence of cerebro-vascular disease has been reported to be high among Japanese people (Kagan *et al*, 1976).

Dementia and depression

Depression occurs in the context of dementia (Alexopoulos & Abrams, 1991) and is also a risk factor for dementia (e.g. Reynolds *et al*, 1986), particularly late-onset Alzheimer's disease (Breteler *et al*, 1992). This is true of depression occurring at least 10 years prior to the onset of dementia, implying a causal association. Possible mechanisms include common neurochemical aetiology, an effect of antidepressant medication and a lowering of the threshold for dementia detection caused by subtle cognitive impairments in depression (Breteler *et al*, 1992).

The association between dementia and depression can present a diagnostic difficulty. As Alexopoulos & Abrams (1991) point out, a distinction should be made between depression–dementia syndromes and depression related to behavioural disturbances in dementia. However, depression itself is a complex construct in a cross-cultural setting. This places great demands on the clinician to make adequate differential diagnoses when both depression and dementia are present in such a setting. Depression should, therefore, be considered in detail.

Depression

Much cross-cultural psychiatric research has involved the application of instruments and of disease categories, devised from decades of work with European and American patients, to samples of people from different cultures. This method, coined the 'etic' approach by anthropologists, assumes that disorders such as depression have universal validity, an assumption which has been the focus of increasing debate in recent years (Littlewood, 1990; also see Chapters 4 and 5). Etic studies take instruments developed in one setting, then translate and apply them with little or no modification to another culture. 'Emic' studies, in contrast, are qualitative, relatively rare and attempt to generate rich descriptions of symptoms and of behaviour within a specific culture (Manson *et al*, 1985; Beiser, 1985; see Chapter 5).

While there is evidence to support the existence of broad similarities in the pattern of depression across cultures (Marsella *et al*, 1985), there are also differences, particularly in the expression and experience of the more common but less severe forms of depression and anxiety (Beiser, 1985; Kleinman, 1987; Abas & Broadhead, 1997). As well as evidence that people may somatically express and experience distress more often in some cultures than in others, it has been suggested that sadness may overlap more with anxiety and irritability in some societies (Leff, 1988). Others have argued that 'core' features of depression may have different cross-cultural meanings (Obeyesekere, 1985) and that syndromes of emotional distress are better understood by some as disturbances of 'the soul' rather than as mental depression (Kleinman, 1987).

The 'new cross-cultural psychiatry' (Kleinman, 1977) aims to combine etic and emic approaches, but as yet its methodology remains lengthy, complex and unresolved (Patel *et al*, 1997). The first stage of this methodology involves reviewing the ethnographic literature for the culture to be studied and interviewing those who, in that culture, are principally involved in the treatment of the mentally ill at a community level, such as religious healers. From this, it is possible to define concepts of mental illness and terminology in common use for emotional distress. Patients identified by care providers working from within the culture can be interviewed to elicit emic and etic phenomenology (Abas *et al*, 1996). Symptom profiles derived from both sources can shed light on the presentation of common mental disorders in the community, and a screening instrument can be developed and used for clinical and research purposes.

Screening and cross-cultural assessment of depression in the UK

One stereotype that has served to retard psychiatric research and service development for ethnic minority elders is the perception that they overwhelmingly somatise depression. This misconception may be linked to 'colonial' inability to admit the range of emotions experienced by people of African and Asian descent and to lack of enquiry beyond the somatic facade (Weiss & Kleinman, 1988). In contrast, we have found that Black Caribbean elders (for example) use a very rich psychological language to describe states of stress and lowering of spirit. In a recent pilot community study (Richards *et al*, 1996) we found that 17% of a random sample of Caribbean elders had notable emotional distress, although only half of these met psychiatric diagnostic criteria for depression (DSM–III–R; American Psychiatric Association, 1987). Of those significantly distressed but not meeting DSM–III–R criteria, two-thirds were recognised by their families and by a Caribbean nurse to be severely 'stressed' and in need of help. All had unmet needs (e.g. assistance with caring for a spouse with dementia, assessment of physical illness, prescription of antidepressants). Many of these were subsequently addressed through existing health and social care provision but some services offered were seen by elders and their families as inappropriate . These findings raise questions about: (a) whether screening tools and diagnostic criteria for depression, validated in White subjects, are fully adequate for use with ethnic minority elders; and (b) to what extent are the needs of depressed subjects being met and, if they are not, how could services be improved?

The Geriatric Depression Scale (GDS; Yesavage, 1988) was specifically developed for screening for emotional distress in the elderly and is now recommended by the Royal College of General Practitioners. However, it has not been validated in older people from the larger ethnic minority groups. Instruments can give misleading estimates when used in other cultures unless they are first validated for those cultures. It will be crucial to test whether the GDS is 'culture-fair' in older people from other cultural groups, that is, whether the recommended cut-off leads to under- or overestimation of emotional distress, relative to the White population (D'Ath *et al*, 1994).

Development of a preliminary culture-specific screen for emotional distress for use with Black Caribbean elders

A study currently in progress in south-east London will be described to illustrate the application of some aspects of the new cross-cultural psychiatry. A combination of semi-structured interviews with non-psychiatrically trained carers for elderly Black Caribbean people (including church ministers, voluntary workers, practice nurses and home care organisers) and with elders identified by those workers as emotionally distressed has been used to generate a lay Caribbean classification of mental illness categories. Techniques used were adapted from a range of anthropological and psychiatric studies (Kleinman, 1980; Wig *et al*, 1980; Manson *et al*, 1985; Khan & Manderson, 1992). Many of those interviewed held a unitary view of mental disorder and stress as the end result of a variety of insults. Severe insults and/or 'inability to cope with stress' would lead to 'a stressful condition/depression of the spirit/depression' and this could deteriorate to states of 'confusion' and of 'not making sense' (Abas *et al*, 1996).

Over 100 idioms, apparently linked to non-psychotic distress, were collected. Depression was mentioned by only 9% of respondents and suicide by none. A consensus approach was used to group the idioms into domains, 11 domains emerging as particularly dominant, for example: worrying/fretting; feeling low or down; feeling pressured; feeling empty inside; being weighed down; feeling cut-off or alone. An idiom from one of these domains was mentioned by 15–63% of respondents. These 11 key domains were thus chosen to create a preliminary Caribbean culture-specific screen (PCSS; see Box 1).

Compared with scales recommended for detection among White British subjects (Bird *et al*, 1987; Yesavage, 1988) there is some overlap in terms concerning poor sleep, worry and lack of energy/tiredness. However there are also some differences. The Caribbean term 'feeling cut-off' may reflect heightened feelings of social or family alienation (Sokolovsky, 1990) or of loss of a homeland (Manthorp & Hettiaratchy, 1993) but neither that term nor the common expression of 'feeling fed-up' feature on the other standard scales. Whereas the question on emptiness in the GDS is connected

---

Box 1
Items in the preliminary culture-specific screen PCSS for emotional distress in Caribbean elders

In the past month:

1. Have you been worrying too much or fretting?
2. Have you felt pressured, like pressure is rising in the head?
3. Have you had lots of pain or gas in the belly or the pit of your stomach?
4. What about pain or aching all over the body?
5. Have you felt weak or tired?
6. Have you slept well?
7. Have you been feeling down or low spirited or like you're crying inside?
8. Have you felt fed up with yourself or even with others, like you want to curse or scream?
9. Have you felt cut-off or alone, or been feeling empty or spiritless inside?
10. Do you feel weighed down by life?
11. Do you still feel hopeful?

---

with life being empty, those questioned here emphasised emptiness or spiritlessness as emerging from inside themselves. A tendency for people of Caribbean origin to feel low rather than depressed or sad, and to complain of tiredness and diffuse pain when depressed, has also been described in older African American people in Baltimore (Baker *et al*, 1995). Other features of this scale include items possibly linked to anxiety and tension such as feeling pressured and having a sensation of gas bubbling in the stomach. It is thus likely that this scale will be sensitive in detecting the common forms of depressive disorder seen in primary care, given their common association with anxiety.

Pilot validation has been carried out in Caribbean elders from a community and a clinical sample, most of whom were born in Jamaica. The screen performed well in discriminating between depressed cases and non-depressed cases, with a sensitivity and specificity above 80% at a cut-off of 4/5. However, the criteria for caseness were based on a medical psychiatric assessment and, as Helman (1990) has outlined, mental disorder should be defined within parameters agreed as abnormal by key people from one's own culture. A full-scale validation of the PCSS and the GDS will thus require two sets of validating criteria, one being a standardised psychiatric interview (Copeland *et al*, 1986) and the other a culture-specific diagnosis of emotional disorder (Beiser, 1985; Leff, 1990; Helman, 1990). The latter will be based on a consensus between a Black Caribbean psychiatric social worker and a Black Caribbean church minister, both with extensive experience of working with elderly people from the Caribbean region (Abas *et al*, 1998). Statistical modelling can be used to examine the relationship between the two screens and the two sets of validating criteria and to determine the most sensitive and specific screening items (Dunn, 1989). Although there could be similarities in performance between the culture-specific screen and the GDS, it is hypothesised that certain items from the former will enhance detection.

A validated screening tool can thus be developed (possibly combining items from the GDS with items from the PCSS) for use as a case-finding instrument in primary care, for further research which seeks to identify unmet need among depressed Caribbean elders and to improve service delivery. Similar approaches should be used to develop and validate screening instruments for older people from other ethnic minority groups and to clarify key terms that may be indicative of significant depression and anxiety.

Service delivery and unmet need

Although there is increasing professional consensus about the assessment and management of depressive and dementing disorders (Jacoby & Oppenheimer, 1991; Goldberg & Huxley, 1992; Jenkins, 1992; Paykel & Priest, 1992), general practitioners are unlikely to offer such treatment to elderly people from ethnic minorities and experience particular difficulty in assessing mental ill health in people from these groups (Lloyd, 1993; Pharaoh, 1994). The limited data available suggest that, like the children, ethnic minority elders are under-represented among patients in touch with National Health Service community and hospital mental health facilities (Bahl, 1993; Pharoah, 1994; Abas, 1996). There could be many reasons for this, including a genuinely lower prevalence of disorders, as has been suggested for depression by some studies in the USA (Gibson, 1988; Blazer, 1990) and for dementia, or failure of medical staff to realise the significance of terminology in common use. The impression, however, is that other factors are of crucial importance, including lack of awareness of and/or a negative perception of statutory services, documented elsewhere with respect to low uptake of home help and community nursing provision (Norman, 1985). If services are to be made more accessible and appropriate, it will be vital to study attitudes towards depression and dementia and towards acceptable service provision and to compare differences between consulters and non-consulters. Although professional estimates of need, met and unmet, can be valuable, consumer and family expectations and opinions must be sought (Slade, 1994).

The explanatory model approach (Kleinman, 1980; Helman, 1990; Weiss *et al*, 1992; discussed in Chapter 7) can be used to explore the person's own notions about an episode of sickness and its appropriate treatment and can also gather information about cultural background and experience in the host culture. This should be extended for the elderly person and, if possible, a family member, to define key problems faced, followed by a systematic enquiry about potential difficulties (e.g. physical, psychological, activities of daily living, relationships, housing), current support and services received, key requirements and attitudes to relevant health and social care treatments, including counselling for psychosocial problems, psychotropic medication, measures to improve isolation and assistance with activities of daily living and how and by whom they should be delivered. By comparing the type and the cost of services being used with similar data for services delivered in the way people would prefer, we can begin to define better packages of care and their full cost implications. Preferences may not all involve great financial costs.

Although specific services, for example, counselling provided by Black staff, may be preferable, pilot interviews suggest that a sense of being listened to, by someone of any nationality, will help to overcome perceived barriers. Pilot interviews have also indicated the need for awareness of and a non-judgmental attitude towards cultural differences, such as variations in family structures, the tendency for older people to bring up young grandchildren and the discomfort in accepting help from outside agencies. A professional's readiness to acknowledge and discuss factors operating for the patient (such as racism and deprivation) is fundamental, and referral to voluntary, religious, community health and local authority services should be welcomed. In this cultural group, pilot interviews suggest that lay theories of mental disorders in older people from some ethnic minorities centre around them being secondary to a variety of unmet needs (including physical, social and spiritual), hence it would be culturally offensive to focus on the diagnosis of mental illness without an exploration of wider requirements for care.

Conclusions

The emphasis of provision of health services in a multiracial, multicultural society demands that the National Health Service can respond to the diversity of need. The evidence we have presented seeks to emphasise that it is only through respect of differences in the presentation, assessment and management of common mental disorders among older people from different cultures, through the integration of qualitative and quantitative research methods and through training and dissemination of information that existing services can become truly responsive to the requirements of a rich and varied population.

Acknowledgements

This chapter was prepared during an Alzheimer's Disease Society Research Fellowship to M.R.

References

ABAS, M. A. (1996) Depression and anxiety among older African–Caribbean people in the UK: screening, unmet need and the provision of appropriate services. *International Journal of Geriatric Psychiatry*, **11**, 377–382.

——, PHILLIPS, C., RICHARDS, M., *et al* (1996) Initial development of a new culture-specific screen for emotional distress in older African–Caribbean people. *International Journal of Geriatric Psychiatry*, **11**, 1097–1103.

—— & BROADHEAD, J. C. (1997) Depression and anxiety among women in an urban setting in Zimbabwe. *Psychological Medicine*, **27**, 59–71.

——, PHILLIPS, C., CARTER, J., *et al* (1998) Culturally sensitive validation of screening questionnaires for depression in older African–Caribbean people living in south London. *British Journal of Psychiatry*, **173**, 249–254.

ALEXOPOULOS, G. S. & ABRAMS, R. C. (1991) Depression in Alzheimer's disease. *Psychiatric Clinics of North America*, **14**, 327–340.

AMERICAN HEART ASSOCIATION (1995) *Heart and Stroke Facts: 1995 Statistical Supplement*. Dallas, TX: American Heart Association.

AMERICAN PSYCHIATRIC ASSOCIATION (1980) *Diagnostic and Statistical Manual of Mental Disorders.* (DSM–III) (3rd edn). Washington, DC: APA.

—— (1987) *Diagnostic and Statistical Manual of Mental Disorders* (DSM–III–R) (3rd edn, revised). Washington, DC: APA.

—— (1994) *Diagnostic and Statistical Manual of Mental Disorders* (DSM–IV) (4th edn). Washington, DC: APA.

BAHL, V. (1993) Access to health care for Black and ethnic minority elderly people: general principles. In *Access to Health Care for People from Black and Ethnic Minorities* (eds A. Hopkins & V. Bahl), pp. 93–97. London: Royal College of Physicians of London.

BAKER, F. M., PARKER, D. A., WILEY, C., *et al* (1995) Depressive symptoms in African American medical patients. *International Journal of Geriatric Psychiatry*, **10**, 9–14.

BEISER, M. (1985) A study of depression among traditional Africans, urban North Americans, and Southeast Asian refugees. In *Culture and Depression* (eds A. Kleinman & B. Good), pp. 272–298. Berkeley, CA: University of California Press.

BIRD, A. S., MACDONALD, A. J. D., MANN, A. H., *et al* (1987) Preliminary experience with the SELFCARE (D): A self-rating depression questionnaire for use in elderly, non-institutionalised subjects. *International Journal of Geriatric Psychiatry*, **2**, 31–38.

BLAZER, D. G. (1990) Life events, mental health functioning and the use of healthcare services by the elderly. *American Journal of Public Health*, **10**, 1174–1179.

BRETELER, M. M. B., CLAUS, J. J., VAN DUIJN, C. M., *et al* (1992) Epidemiology of Alzheimer's disease. *Epidemiologic Reviews*, **14**, 59–82.

CHANDRA, V., GANGULI, M., RATCLIFF, G., *et al* (1994) Studies of the epidemiology of dementia: comparisons between developed and developing countries. *Aging and Clinical Experimental Research*, **6**, 307–321.

——, ——, ——, *et al* (1999) Practical issues in cognitive screening of elderly populations in developing countries – the Indo–US National Dementia Epidemiology Study. *Aging and Clinical Experimental Research*, in press.

COPELAND, J. R., DEWEY, M. E. & GRIFFITHS-JONES, H. M. (1986) A computerised psychiatric diagnostic system and case nomenclature for elderly subjects: GMS and AGECAT. *Psychological Medicine*, **16**, 89–99.

D'ATH, P., MULLAN, N., KATONA, P., *et al* (1994) Screening, detection and management of depression in elderly primary care attenders. I. The acceptability and performance of 15-item Geriatric Depression Scale (GDS–15) and the development of shorter versions. *Family Practice*, **11**, 260–266.

DE LA MONTE, S. M., HUTCHINS, G. M. & MOORE, G. (1989) Racial differences in the etiology of dementia and frequency of Alzheimer lesions in the brain. *Journal of the National Medical Association*, **81**, 644–652.

DUNN, G. (1989) *Design and Analysis of Reliability Studies: Statistical Evaluation of Measurement Errors*. London: Edward Arnold.

FILLENBAUM, G. G., CHANDRA, V., GANGULI, M., *et al* (1999) Development of an Activities of Daily Living Scale for an illiterate rural older population in India. *Age and Aging*, in press.

GIBSON, R. C. (1988) Aging in Black America: the effects of an aging society. In *Aging in Cross-Cultural Perspective* (ed. E. Gort), pp. 105–129. New York: Phelps-Stokes Fund.

GOLDBERG, D. & HUXLEY, P. (1992) *Common Mental Disorders: A Bio-Social Model*. London: Routledge.

HELMAN, C. G. (1990) *Culture, Health and Illness* (2nd edn). Bristol: Wright.

HENDERSON, A. S. (1986) The epidemiology of Alzheimer's disease. *British Medical Bulletin*, **42**, 3–10.

HENDRIE, H. C., OSTUNTOKUN, B. O., HALL, K. S., *et al* (1995) Prevalence of Alzheimer's disease and dementia in two communities: Nigerian Africans and African Americans. *American Journal of Psychiatry*, **152**, 1485–1492.

HEYMAN, A., FILLENBAUM, G., PROSNITZ, B., *et al* (1991) Estimated prevalence of dementia among elderly Black and White community residents. *Archives of Neurology*, **48**, 594–598.

HOFMAN, A., ROCCA, W. A., BRAYNE, C., *et al* (1991) The prevalence of dementia in Europe: a collaborative study of 1980–1990 findings. *International Journal of Epidemiology*, **20**, 736–748.

JACOBY, R. & OPPENHEIMER, C. (eds) (1991) *Psychiatry in the Elderly*. Oxford: Oxford University Press.

JENKINS, R. (1992) Health targets. In *Measuring Mental Health Needs* (eds G. Thornicroft, C. R. Brewin & J. Wing), pp. 18–41. London: Gaskell.

JORM, A. F. (1990) *The Epidemiology of Alzheimer's Disease and Related Disorders*. London: Chapman and Hall.

KAGAN, A., POPPER, J., RHOADS, G. G., *et al* (1976) Epidemiological studies of coronary heart disease and stroke in Japanese men living in Japan, Hawaii, and California: prevalence of stroke. In *Cerebrovascular Diseases* (ed. P. Scheinberg). Raven Press: New York.

KHAN, M. E. & MANDERSON, L. (1992) Focus groups in tropical diseases research. *Health Policy and Planning*, **7**, 56–66.

KLEINMAN, A. (1977) Depression, somatisation and the "new cross-cultural psychiatry". *Social Science and Medicine*, **11**, 3–10.

—— (1980) *Patients and Healers in the Context of Culture*. London: University of California Press.

—— (1987) Anthropology and psychiatry: the role of culture in cross-cultural research on illness. *British Journal of Psychiatry*, **151**, 447–454.

LEFF, J. (1988) *Psychiatry Around the Globe* (2nd edn). London: Gaskell.
—— (1990) The "new cross-cultural psychiatry": a case of the baby and the bathwater. *British Journal of Psychiatry*, **156**, 305–307.
LI, G., SHEN, Y. C., CHEN, C. H., *et al* (1989) An epidemiological survey of age-related dementia in an urban area of Beijing. *Acta Psychiatrica Scandinavica*, **79**, 557–563.
LITTLEWOOD, R. (1990) From categories to contexts: a decade of the 'new cross-cultural psychiatry'. *British Journal of Psychiatry*, **156**, 308–327.
LLOYD, K. (1993) Depression and anxiety among Afro-Caribbean general practice attenders in Britain. *International Journal of Social Psychiatry*, **39**, 1–9.
McKHANN, G., DRACHMAN, D., FOLSTEIN, M., *et al* (1984) Clinical diagnosis of Alzheimer's disease: report of the NINCDS–ADRDA Work Group under the auspices of Department of Health and Human Services Task Force on Alzheimer's Disease. *Neurology*, **34**, 939–944.
MANSON, S. M., SHORE, J. H. & BLOOM, J. D. (1985) The depressive experience in American Indian Communities: A challenge for psychiatric theory and diagnosis. In *Culture and Depression* (eds A. Kleinman & B. Good), pp. 331–368. Berkley, CA: University of California Press.
MANTHORP, E. J. & HETTIARATCHY, P. (1993) Ethnic minority elders in the UK. *International Review of Psychiatry*, **5**, 171–178.
MARSELLA, A. J., SARTORIUS, N., JABLENSKY, A. *et al* (1985) Cross-cultural studies of depression. In *Culture and Depression* (eds A. Kleinman & B. Good), pp. 299–324. Berkeley, CA: University of California Press.
MILLER, D., HICKS, S. P., D'AMATO, C. J., *et al* (1984) A descriptive study of neurotic plaques and neurofibrillary tangles in an autopsy population. *American Journal of Epidemiology*, **120**, 331–341.
NATIONAL HEART, LUNG AND BLOOD INSTITUTE (1995) Hypertension prevalence and the status of awareness, treatment and control in the United States. *Hypertension*, **7**, 457–468.
NORMAN, A. (1985) *Triple Jeopardy: Growing Old in a Second Homeland*. London: Centre for Policy on Ageing.
OBEYESEKERE, G. (1985) Depression, Buddhism and the work of culture in Sri Lanka. In *Culture and Depression* (eds A. Kleinman & B. Good), pp. 134–152. Berkeley, CA: University of California Press.
OGUNNIYI, A. O., OSUNTOKUN, B. O., LEWAUKA, U. B., *et al* (1992) Rarity of dementia (by DSM–III–R) in an urban community in Nigeria. *East African Medical Journal*, **69**, 64–68.
OSUNTOKUN, B. O., ADEUJA, A. O. G., SCHOENBERG, B. S., *et al* (1987) Neurological disorders in Nigerian Africans: a community-based study. *Acta Neurologica Scandinavica*, **75**, 13–21.
——, OGUNNIYI, A. O., LEKWAUWA, U. G., *et al* (1990) Epidemiology of dementia in Nigerian Africans. In *Advances in Neurology* (eds J. S. Chopra, K. Jagannathan & I. M. S. Sawhney), pp. 331–342. Amsterdam: Excerpta Medica.
——, HENDRIE, H. C., OGUNNIYI, A. O., *et al* (1992) Cross-cultural studies in Alzheimer's disease. *Ethnicity and Disease*, **2**, 352–357.
——, OGUNNIYI, A., AKANG, E. E. U., *et al* (1994) A4-amyloid in the brains of non-demented Nigerian Africans. *Lancet*, **343**, 56.
PATEL, V., GWANZURA, F., SIMUNYU, E., *et al* (1997) The phenomenology and explanatory models of common mental disorder: a study in primary care in Harare, Zimbabwe. *Psychological Medicine*, **25**, 1191–1199.
PAYKEL, E. S. & PRIEST, R. G. (1992) Recognition and management of depression in general practice: consensus statement. *British Medical Journal*, **305**, 1198–1202.
PHARAOH, C. (1994) *The Provision of Primary Health Care for Elderly People from Black and Minority Ethnic Communities*. London: Age Concern, Institute of Gerontology, King's College.
REYNOLDS, C. F., KUMPFER, D. J., HOCH, C. C., *et al* (1986) Two-year follow-up of elderly patients with mixed depression and dementia. Clinical and electrencephalographic sleep findings. *Journal of the American Geriatric Society*, **34**, 793–799.

RICHARDS, M. & CHAUDHURI, R. K. (1996) Parkinson's disease in populations of African origin: a review of the literature. *Neuroepidemiology*, **15**, 214–221.

——, BRAYNE, C., FORDE, C., *et al* (1996) Surveying African-Caribbean elders in the community: implications for research on health and health service use. *Internationl Journal of Psychogeriatrics*, **11**, 41–45.

SCHOENBERG, B. S., ANDERSON, D. W. & HAERER, A. F. (1985) Severe dementia: prevalence and clinical features in a biracial US population. *Archives of Neurology*, **42**, 740–743.

SIEGEL, J. S. & HOOVER, S. L. (1982) Demographic aspects of the health of the elderly to the year 2000 and beyond. *World Health Statistics Quarterly*, **46**, 91–96.

SLADE, M. (1994) Needs assessment. *British Journal of Psychiatry*, **165**, 293–296.

SOKOLOVSKY, J. (1990) *The Cultural Context of Ageing*. New York: Bergin and Garvey.

STILL, C. N., JACKSON, K. L., BRANDES, D. A., *et al* (1990) Distribution of major dementias by race and sex in South Carolina. *Journal of the South Carolina Medical Association*, **86**, 453–456.

TREVES, T., KORCZYN, A. D., ZILBER, N., *et al* (1986) Presenile dementia in Israel. *Archives of Neurology*, **43**, 26–29.

VAN DUIJN, C. M., STIJNEN, T. & HOFMAN, A. (1991) Risk factors for Alzheimer's disease: overview of the EURODEM collaborative re-analysis of case-control studies. *International Journal of Epidemiology*, **20** (suppl. 2).

WEISS, M. G. & KLEINMAN, A. (1988) Depression in cross-cultural perspective: developing a culturally informed model. In *Health and Cross-Cultural Psychology* (eds P. R. Dasen, J. W. Berry & N. Sartorius). Newbury Park, CA: Sage Publications.

——, DOONGAJI, D. R., SIDDHARTHA, S., *et al* (1992) The Explanatory Model Interview Catalogue (EMIC). Contribution to cross-cultural research methods from a study of leprosy and mental health. *British Journal of Psychiatry*, **160**, 819–830.

WIG, N. N., SULEIMAN, M. A., ROUTLEDGE, R., *et al* (1980) Community reactions to mental disorders: a key informant study in three developing countries. *Acta Psychiatrica Scandinavica*, **61**, 111–126.

WORLD HEALTH ORGANIZATION (1980) *The International Classification of Impairments, Disabilities, and Handicaps*. Geneva: WHO.

—— (1992) *The Tenth Revision of the International Classification of Diseases and Related Health Problems* (ICD–10). Geneva: WHO.

YESAVAGE, G. A. (1988) Geriatric Depression Scale. *Psychopharmacology Bulletin*, **24**, 709–710.

ZHANG, M., KATZMAN, R., SALMON, D., *et al* (1990) The prevalence of dementia and Alzheimer's disease in Shanghai, China: impact of age, gender, and education. *Annals of Neurology*, **27**, 428–437.

12 Suicide and attempted suicide across cultures

DINESH BHUGRA, MANISHA DESAI and DAVID BALDWIN

Suicide and attempted suicide have existed since time immemorial and both phenomena have puzzled clinicians and scientists alike. The reasons for these acts are often unclear, especially if the historical aspects of attempted and completed suicide are studied. As Van Hooff (1994) suggests, in ancient (European) cultures suicide was common and he reports that, according to historical documents, women preferred to hang themselves as a method of suicide, whereas men used tools for stabbing and cutting. Self-poisoning was not common. The methods demonstrate the resoluteness of the person who had decided to put an end to his or her life. In ancient Hindu texts (Vedic period 4000–2000 BC) killing oneself was allowed, but in the later Uprishadic period suicide was condemned even though it was still acceptable for the *sanyasis* (holy people) who had gained insight into their being and the universe. Suicide was permitted on religious grounds, as death could offer an opportunity for a new beginning (Venkoba Rao, 1981). For the Indian woman, *suttee* (killing herself when her husband died) was voluntary initially, but later became obligatory. There are accounts of mass suicide by women burning themselves or jumping into wells (*jauhar*) in the Rajputana regions, especially if they wanted to avoid humiliation and molestation by invading armies. Hunger strikes or self-immolation for political causes are well known in the Indian context.

Definitions

The literature on suicidal behaviour can be divided into suicide and attempted suicide or parasuicide, which has also been equated with deliberate self-harm. Diekstra (1994) suggests that many parasuicidal behaviours differ from suicide in demographic, social, functional and behavioural characteristics.

The term suicide commonly refers to any death that is the direct or indirect result of a positive or negative act accomplished by the victim which the victim knows will produce the desired result. This definition obviously implies that the term suicide should be applied only in cases of death, and that intentional risk-taking leading to death is also suicide; Diekstra (1994) points out that the latter is a common but neglected form of suicide.

Parasuicide covers behaviours that are suicidal gestures or manipulative attempts at help-seeking or unsuccessful attempts to kill oneself. The act should be non-habitual and is usually carried out at the height of a crisis.

Some confusion remains over the use of these terms in different countries. They may or may not clarify the intent. Assessment should always cover the intent as well as the behaviour. A considerable range exists between the two behaviours and indirect suicide or accidental suicide lies somewhere in the middle.

Epidemiological issues

As discussed earlier in Chapters 1 and 4, one of the basic problems in epidemiological studies is the use of definitions. In addition, various countries have different rules and regulations for reporting and monitoring suicide and parasuicide. Where attempted suicide is a criminal offence there is an incentive to label suicidal behaviour as accidental. Furthermore, rates of attempted suicide are often collected from hospital data, which makes estimates of incidence rates problematic. The hospital data for parasuicide are often administrative and may not give a clue to the intent or whether distress was being expressed in any psychological way. In addition, entry to the hospital system depends very much on the health care system, availability of services and attitudes of the casualty staff to parasuicide. Thus, international comparisons of rates are problematic. Even within the same country there may be regional variations which may not be explained by simple socio-demographic variables.

Parasuicide has generated more interest than suicide in Europe and two international studies have been carried out. However, neither of these looked at ethnicity. There is clear evidence that parasuicide rates vary according to region and gender (see below). Peak ages for parasuicide seem to fall (both in terms of absolute numbers and in rates per 100 000 of the particular age group) within the first half of the life cycle. Diekstra (1985) estimated a crude annual incidence rate of parasuicide from these studies of 300–800 per 100 000 in the population aged 15 years and over. Estimates of one-year prevalence of parasuicidal acts varied from 2.4 to 20% (Dubow *et al*, 1989; Nagy & Adcock, 1990; Centers for Disease Control, 1991) with a lifetime prevalence from 2.2 to 20% (Rubinstein *et al*, 1989; Diekstra *et al*, 1991).

Methods

The methods for suicide and suicide attempts vary with gender and across national divides. For suicide, males are more likely to use violent means like hanging, shooting, jumping off tall buildings and traffic or train injuries, whereas females are more likely to take poisons. However, it is not always clear from the data whether the means of the attempt were in themselves successful or were precipitants.

The cultural and religious pressures to keep suicidal acts secret, along with legal structures, may mean that the actual method is not clearly revealed. Methods of suicide and parasuicide very much depend upon their availability. In agricultural societies, for example, swallowing organophosphorus compounds is common, whereas in industrialised urban societies the use of car exhaust fumes may be much higher. Ethnicity seems to be related to the choice of substance used in self-poisoning (Mahy, 1993). The choice of means also depends upon any underlying psychiatric illnesses that may exist. Schizophrenia and affective disorder along with substance misuse contribute to high suicide and parasuicide rates in certain countries, usually through self-poisoning.

Gender differences

The relationship of both suicide and attempted suicide with gender and age is well known (Vaillant & Blumenthal, 1990). Suicide risk increases with age. In the first study of attempted suicide across various centres in Europe, Diekstra (1982) observed an average rate of 215 cases per 100 000 persons aged 15 years and older (162 for males and 265 for females). Between countries, rates varied considerably, from 26 to 353 for males, and from 82 to 527 for females. A second study (Platt *et al*, 1992) showed that in Europe high rates of parasuicide were found in Helsinki (414 in 100 000) and the lowest rate (61 in 100 000) was found in

Leiden (The Netherlands) – a ratio in excess of 7:1. For females, the lowest rates were in Leiden and the highest in Pontoise (France); Helsinki showed higher rates for males.

Jack (1992) argues that despite the staggering statistics, gender is largely ignored in both the theoretical discussion and empirical investigation of self-poisoning. He suggests that the distinction between the suicide and attempted suicide may not always be very clear and the boundaries may be blurred. He criticises psychiatrists for labelling non-psychiatrically ill patients as hysterical, manipulative or aggressive – value-laden labels applied to gender as well.

Suicide in an international context

Several countries report increased rates of suicide and parasuicide in people of Indian origin. Regrettably, the majority of the studies are retrospective and the problems noted above regarding the registration of suicide are often not answered. Moreover, ethnicity, which is generally quite difficult to define, is not always very clearly determined or stated.

Countries as diverse as Singapore, Trinidad, Guyana and Surinam have reported high rates of suicidal behaviour in Indian people, especially young women. Haynes (1987) suggests that in the 19th century the rates were high among Indian indentured labourers in Fiji and these were attributed to a low ratio of female to male immigrants, leading to rivalry and jealousy along with feelings of nostalgia and the intense desire to return to India (Tinker, 1974). Similarly in the Caribbean the rates are higher in the countries which have a significant Indo-Caribbean population. Mahy (1993) using World Health Organization statistics reported that Barbados had a suicide rate of 2.8 per 100 000 between 1968 and 1971 with a male to female ratio of 3.8:1. Around the same period the rates in Jamaica were 1.4 and in the Bahamas 2.8. In 1974 the rate in Trinidad and Tobago was 7 per 100 000, which had nearly doubled to 11.9 per 100 000 by 1988. Suicides precipitated by disputes with loved ones or within the family were higher for Indo-Trinidadians (Mahy, 1993). By 1989, the rate in Barbados had gone up to 62 per 100 000 and in St Lucia and Grenada it was 4 per 100 000. For comparison, in the USA, the age-adjusted suicide rate per 100 000 in 1986 was 11.9 (National Center for Health Statistics, 1988).

The prevalence of suicide in Black males (10.5 per 100 000) in the USA is several times higher than it is for Black females (2.2 per

100 000; US Department of Health & Human Services, 1985). The peak rates occur between 20 and 34 years of age. The rates of suicide among Hispanic people in the USA appear to be somewhat lower than those in the White population (Earls *et al*, 1990). In Puerto Rico, the rate of completed suicide has been shown to be 9.2 per 100 000, and has been remarkably stable over 25 years (Earls *et al*, 1990). Among Native Americans and Alaskan Inuit in 1980–1982 the rates were 19.4 per 100 000, 1.7 times higher than the national average; the differences were even greater for younger age groups (May, 1987).

Maniam (1988) reported that suicide rates were highest in the female Indian population in the Cameron highlands of Malaysia. Haynes (1984) observed rates of 71.9 per 100 000 in Indian women in the Macuata province of Fiji compared with national rates of 33.1 per 100 000 among the Indian and 9.3 per 100 000 among the Fijian population. This was based on police records of unnatural deaths that had received verdicts of suicide in the magistrate's court. In a similar study Ree (1971) reported similar findings. However, in Singapore, Peng & Choo (1986) observed that even though the suicide rates were rising in the Indian women, these were still lower than those reported among Chinese women.

On the Indian subcontinent itself, there are marked regional variations in suicide rates – from 2.93 per 100 000 in Delhi to 43 in 100 000 in Madurai. These variations may be due to data being collected at very different times as well as to ethnic variation. Furthermore, since attempting suicide is a criminal offence and because of the existence of dowry deaths (being set on fire by the husband's family demanding larger dowries – often classified as accidents), the true rates may be obscured. Within two different geographical areas of West Bengal, a marked difference in rates has been reported (Adityanjee, 1976): 5.13 per 100 000 and 28.57 per 100 000. Nevertheless, India continues to have lower suicide rates than most Western countries (Venkoba Rao, 1981). In Sri Lanka, suicide rates have increased dramatically, from 9.9 per 100 000 in 1960 (Dissanayake & de Silva, 1981) to the second highest suicide rate among all the countries reporting to the World Health Organization more recently (Le Vachia *et al*, 1994). The rates are higher for Sri Lankan Tamils than the Sinhalese and are lower among women. In Pakistan, the reported rate of suicide was 1.24 per 100 000, which again is an underestimate because of the stigma attached to suicide.

It is apparent that the literature on suicide trends across cultures and countries shows trends and themes which suggest that the following tentative observations can be made.

(a) Suicide rates are higher for Indian men, but in the younger age group it is more common in women.
(b) The rates are generally higher among Asian immigrants than among the native population.
(c) Methods of suicide vary with the local availability of poisonous substances and local customs and cultures.
(d) Self-immolation has been shown to be a cause for higher suicide rates in Indian women.
(e) In the Asian subcontinent, suicidal behaviour is most common among young single females, followed by married women.
(f) Precipitating factors are usually interpersonal difficulties either within the family or within a relationship. Alcohol and financial causes are rarely reported.
(g) The issues of low self-esteem, early marriage, expectations from marriage and family conflicts have not yet been resolved and more work needs to be done in this area.

Attempted suicide in an international context

Attempted suicide has its own difficulties in terms of measurement and the ascertainment of causes. Only one in four parasuicides leads to contact with health services (Diekstra, 1994).

India and the Indian subcontinent

In Madurai in south India between 1974 and 1978 the number of patients presenting with attempted suicide trebled. Of the 114 suicide attempts studied in 1965, 65 were by men (1:0.93) and this male dominance persisted in data collected two years later. The dominant feelings of attempters were depression, anger, spite, jealousy and a desire to get attention. When students were studied 10 years later, 19 out of 35 were male. Twenty were described as hysterical with inadequate or immature personalities, eight had schizophrenia, three were dependent upon drugs, two stammered, one suffered from epilepsy and one had a toxic psychosis. The absence of depression was striking (Venkoba Rao & Chinnian, 1972).

Quarrels with in-laws and interpersonal relationship problems appear to be extremely common causes of attempted suicide (Ponnudurai *et al*,1986; Bannerjee *et al*,1990). Even repeat attempts are linked with alcohol misuse and poor relationships. In a two-year follow-up, Ponnudurai *et al* (1991) found that a sizeable minority could not be traced as a wrong address had been recorded. Of the subjects who were traced, 14% had suicidal intent – men were three times more likely to have suicidal intent than women were. For women, their husbands' unemployment and alcohol misuse were relevant factors.

Ponnudurai *et al* (1986) originally studied 86 patients in Madras and reported that in 10% of cases alcohol had played a significant role and that more than one-third (38%) had made a suicide attempt with organophosphorus compounds. Males were more likely to attempt suicide than females, and the age group 15–20 years was the most vulnerable – a finding confirmed in other studies (Venkoba Rao, 1965; Sathyavathi, 1971). One-quarter of patients had made their suicide attempt following interpersonal difficulties and arguments. Unemployment and alcohol misuse played an important role. Khan & Reza (1998) reported that in Karachi females were more likely to report relationship problems. Nearly one-fifth (19%) took organophosphorus compounds and 62% took benzodiazepines. In more than half the cases (53%) the attempt was due to acute situational reaction. The various explanations put forward for these rates included the role of religion, political climate, crime rates and arranged marriage, with the issue of control implicit in such decisions. Khan & Reza (1998) and Ashraf (1964) reported that 41% and 44% of their samples, respectively, had attempted suicide as a result of family problems.

In Sri Lanka also, organophosphorus agrochemicals were the most common mode of attempted suicide and, like the Indian studies, males were more likely to attempt suicide (Dissanayake & de Silva, 1981). The common patterns of suicide attempts suggest that males are more likely to attempt suicide with organophosphorus poisoning, the peak age being 15–20 years, with family or relationship problems being the most likely cause.

Far East and elsewhere

Sato *et al* (1993) reported that in their study of 102 people in Japan attempting suicide, 43 had used agricultural compounds, with an increased prevalence in June and December – times of harvest. A majority of cases (53.5%) had no psychiatric history and in nearly one-third the precipitating factor was deterioration in interpersonal relationships. In Malaysia and Hong Kong similar patterns emerge. Maniam (1988) reported that in Malaysia 66% of attempted suicides were by taking agricultural poisons and age-specific rates peaked for thosed aged 15–20 years. Interpersonal difficulties were recorded in about 65% of cases. Younger women were the most likely to have these difficulties and were the group most likely to commit suicide. In Hong Kong, Headley (1981) reported that the peak age for attempts was 20–30 years. Recent immigrants had higher suicide rates and 20% of cases reported interpersonal conflicts and economic stresses (Yap, 1958).

In Saudi Arabia, females were more likely to attempt suicide using analgesics and psychotropic drugs. Again, family relationship difficulties were the most important cause, also confirmed in Nigeria by Odejide *et al* (1986). There is no doubt that availability of certain substances and cultural factors affect suicide attempts. For example, in northern Norway snow-wandering has been described as a method for attempted suicide (Nissen & Haggag, 1988) and in Athens jumping from high buildings has been reported (Konataxakis *et al,* 1988).

Indian diaspora

In Malaysia, three-quarters of parasuicides were by Indians, mostly Tamils. Maniam (1988) hypothesises that the ambivalent attitudes of the Hindu religion may account for some of the increased rates. In Fiji, as Haynes (1987) pointed out, paraquat deaths are common, as are the attempts. She argues that the Indians, because of their historical low status and stereotyping, and because they are still a political minority under-represented in government and professional classes, are probably particularly vulnerable to attempted suicide. In Trinidad, similar findings have been reported (Mahy, 1993). Studies in Trinidad have shown that inter-racial relationships and marriages play a very important role in precipitating suicide attempts.

In the UK, one of the earliest studies addressing the epidemiology of attempted suicide among Asian immigrants was that of Burke (1976), who, in a retrospective case note study, observed that crude adjusted rates were twice as high in females than in males, although repeat attempts were infrequent. Agricultural poisons were rarely taken. Overall, the numbers were low compared to the base population. Nearly half (58%) attributed their attempt to inter-personal problems, although a quarter gave no reason at all. The crude adjusted rates in the immigrants in this study were in the middle of the range of rates reported from natives in India and natives in Edinburgh.

In a prospective study from Birmingham a decade later, Merrill & Owens (1986) reported that the picture was beginning to change. All cases admitted to a hospital following attempted suicide over two years were studied. Of 196 Asian patients, 139 were born on the Indian subcontinent, 52 were born in the UK and a few were born in East Africa. Females were almost three times as likely to present with attempted suicide, and were of a younger age group. Females of Asian origin reported marital problems significantly more frequently and many of these problems were due to cultural conflicts. Arranged marriages, rejections of arranged marriages and associated problems were reported as contributory factors in the Asian female sample. Since the researchers were White and male, by their own reckoning they may have missed some important information. Rates among males and females were compared between Asian, West Indian, Irish, Scottish and English samples. The overall annual rates of self-poisoning in the immigrant groups exceeded those of their country of origin. For Asian and West Indian groups, males and older females were under-represented but young females had similar rates to that of the English group (Merrill & Owens, 1988). Whether this can be explained by Cochrane's selection hypothesis (Cochrane 1977, 1983; also see Chapter 6), that where migration is easy less stable individuals may self-select for migration, and raises interesting issues. Furthermore, reasons for migration and associated stress may need to be studied under these circumstances to explain the reasons why suicide is attempted rather than how.

Glover *et al* (1989) analysed patients aged 10–24 years presenting with self-poisoning to the two casualty departments at The London Hospital between 1980 and 1984. There were no reported suicides, but Asian females constituted an excess in terms of attempted suicide compared with the base population. Wright *et al* (1981) also found high rates in Birmingham. On the other hand, small retrospective studies of Asian adolescents in Coventry and Barnsley showed no differences (Biswas, 1990; Handy *et al*, 1991). Merrill & Owen's (1986) study showed low rates of psychiatric illness, personality disorder, alcohol dependency or past attempts. Once again, it was suggested that Asian females attempt suicide more often and are less likely to have psychiatric problems and more likely to have a history of family and interpersonal conflict.

Nazroo (1997) reported from his community survey of minority ethnic groups that suicidal thoughts were broadly similar across Asian Indian and White groups and these were, surprisingly, lowest in the young, suggesting that the attempts are more likely to be impulsive.

Aetiological factors

In addition to the factors mentioned above which contribute to the causation of suicide attempts, the following are of crucial importance in understanding cross-cultural differences.

Gender roles

Female 'suicide proneness' has been reported as the "self-destructive consequences of sex-role socialisation" (Clifton & Lee, 1976). Jack (1992) argues that in the West (at least) the analogy drawn between the 19th-century epidemic of female hysteria and that of self-poisoning has historical, theoretical and clinical justification. Since the fluctuations in the role of hysteria have paralleled women's domestic and social role changes, it is likely that similar factors are involved for deliberate self-harm. Changes in the cultural milieu but with cultural expectations remaining the same mean that gender role expectations are important. An individual female's expectations of her own gender role, conflicting with the one that she may have been brought up with, and with others' expectations of her, may lead to a dissonance which for other reasons may be unbridgeable. There have been some suggestions (Kessler & McRae, 1983) that the convergence in the ratio of male:female suicidal behaviour is due to increasing occupation by women of non-traditional gender roles. Obviously in societies and cultures where such a theoretical possibility exists, but practical possibilities (for changing gender role expectations or gender role socialisation) are limited or non-existent, a conflict may arise. There have also been suggestions by Kessler & McRae (1983) that when confronted with problems in family and relationship spheres, women in traditional roles rely on other people for emotional support and do not know how to garner help when this is not available, thereby conforming to a 'learned helplessness' model. Financial and economic dependence and social role dependence in some cultures make any other escape impossible and attempted suicide may be one idiom of distress that is easy to follow.

Availability of method

From this necessarily brief overview, it would appear that the ease with which a method is available will be an important factor in the success of the suicide attempt. There is no doubt that there must be a link between suicidal intent and attempt related to the method which will be used. In rural or agricultural settings, access to agricultural poisons means that the inherent risk is greater. However, in countries like India and Pakistan where a lot of drugs can be bought over the counter, their ingestion can be common. In Surinam, before 1979, hanging and ingestion of undiluted acetic acid were common, but the government then banned the sale of the latter and by 1983 the most common method had changed to ingestion of paraquat (Mahy, 1993). On the Indian subcontinent, self-immolation is not an uncommon cause.

The use of paraquat or paracetamol in attempted overdoses means that preventive measures could include combining these with suitable antidotes.

The relationship of ethnicity and social class with methods of attempted suicide needs to be monitored closely. It is likely that religion could play some role in the method chosen. In addition the role of alcohol needs to be studied in conjunction with the method itself.

Psychiatric illness

The association of psychiatric illness and suicidal behaviour is not always very clear, especially in relation to attempted suicide. As is apparent from the literature, the association is vague in attempted suicide but much clearer for suicide. In cases of attempted suicide, the rates of affective disorder have been shown to be extremely variable across cultures (from 14% in India to 58% in The Netherlands). Similarly, the use of alcohol and underlying organic causes make the variability even greater. There is no doubt that the underlying psychological state needs to be assessed thoroughly but the emphasis has to be on why the attempt was made. It is important to understand the psychopathology as well as gaining a clear cultural and social focus on the act.

Future research

The ethnicity and cultural backgrounds of the individual remain useful starting points for understanding the motives behind attempted suicide. There is some suggestion that, in the USA, this is a leading cause of premature death (Earls *et al*, 1990). The impact of migration and socio-economic and often political disadvantage can contribute to the element of stress. This, combined with a feeling of alienation from the individual's own culture, indicates that their sense of belonging and acceptance is poor, leading to lack of self-esteem which may then lead to minor affective illness. This interlinking needs to be studied in greater detail and newer models of interaction developed. In countries where health care is expensive, the ongoing psychological support may be limited, thereby contributing to risk of repeat suicide attempts. Cultural beliefs, attitudes and explanatory models also contribute to help-seeking, as well as perceptions of the act.

Thus, both majority and minority groups need to be studied. The views of the community will aid the formulation of preventive strategies. In addition, with increased assimilation or cultural identification with the majority culture, features may be inculcated which will enable social scientists along with clinicians to study the causation and impact of suicidal behaviour.

Another area which has received scant attention in cultural contexts is that of the relationship between ideators, attempters and completers. It is conceivable that different factors work at different levels within the three groups. As the ideators can belong to any age group, the attempters are younger and the completers are male and older, a theoretical model for preventive strategies begins to emerge. However, the association between these three groups and their relationship with other factors would need to be studied closely. Suicidal behaviour needs to be studied across the life cycle and also in relationship to gender roles, to power relationships between males and females, to cultural and social expectations and to individuals' functioning and expectations. Pharmacological treatments for minor affective disorders must be evaluated thoroughly.

Conclusions

There is no doubt that suicidal behaviours are complex, with a marked interaction between personal, psychological, biological, social and cultural factors. The individual's relationship with his or her own culture and with the social support system is vital in working out a defence strategy.

The available literature suggests that there is an excess of attempted suicide in some ethnic groups, which has been linked with an element of culture conflict producing a cognitive dissonance between the individual and his or her social environment. Feelings of powerlessness, hopelessness and hostility may contribute to increasing rates. Even when outward expression of hostility is possible and acceptable, the individual may direct it inwards, thereby making suicidal attempt more likely. Easy availability of certain methods means that the individual will attempt suicide with whatever is accessible. There remain gender and culture differences between the characteristics of ideators, attempters and completers, and clinicians need to be aware of the differences and if and how the three groups can represent a continuum of suicidal behaviour. As relationship problems take on an important role, the role of the family, its perceptions of the act and its role in supporting the individual become major issues.

It would appear from the available information that certain groups and individuals are more prone to suicidal behaviour, but the underlying factors are not always very clear. The aims of the clinician and the researcher must include unravelling these underlying reasons so that appropriate preventive strategies can be developed.

References

ADITYANJEE, (1976) Suicide attempts and suicides in India: cross cultural aspects. *International Journal of Social Psychiatry*, **32**, 64–73.

ASHRAF, M. (1964) The problem of suicide in Karachi. *Pakistan Armed Forces Medical Journal*, **14**, 156–167.

BANNERJEE, G., NANDI, D., NANDI, S., *et al* (1990) The vulnerability of Indian women to suicide: a field study. *Indian Journal of Psychiatry*, **32**, 305–308.

BISWAS, S. (1990) Ethnic differences in self-poisoning: a comparative study between an Asian and White adolescent group. *Journal of Adolescence*, **13**, 189–193.

BURKE, A. W. (1976) Attempted suicide among Asian immigrants in Birmingham. *British Journal of Psychiatry*, **128**, 528–533.

CENTERS FOR DISEASE CONTROL (1991) Attempted suicide among high school students – US 1990. *Journal of American Medical Association*, **266**, 911.

CLIFTON, A. & LEE, D. (1976) Self-destructive consequences of sex-role socialisation. *Suicidal and Life Threatening Behaviour*, **6**, 1.

COCHRANE, R. (1977) Mental illness in immigrants to England and Wales: an analysis of mental hospital admissions. *Social Psychiatry*, **12**, 25–35.

—— (1983) *The Social Creation of Mental Illness*. London: Longman.

DIEKSTRA, R. F. (1982) Epidemiology of attempted suicide in the EEC. In *New Trends in Suicide Prevention* (eds J. Wilmotte & J. Mendlewicz). Basel: Bibliotheca Psychiatrica.

—— (1985) Suicide and suicide attempts in the European Economic Community. *Suicide and Life Threatening Behaviour*, **15**, 402–421.

—— (1994) On the burden of suicide. In *Divergent Perspectives on Suicidal Behaviour* (ed. M.-J. Kellcher), pp. 2–27. Cork, Ireland: University of Cork.

——, DE HEUS, P., GARNEFSHI, N., *et al* (1991) *Monitoring the Future: Behaviour and Health Among High School Students*. The Hague: NIBUD.

DISSANAYAKE, D. & DE SILVA, P. (1981) Sri Lanka. In *Suicide in Asia and the Near East* (ed. L. Headley), pp. 167–209. Berkeley, CA: University of California Press.

DUBOW, E., KAUSCH, D., BLUM, M., *et al* (1989) Correlates of suicidal ideation and attempts in a community sample of junior high school students. *Journal of Clinical Child Psychology*, **18**, 158–166.

EARLS, F., ESCOBAR, J. & MANSON, S. (1990) Suicide in minority groups: epidemiologic and cultural perspectives. In *Suicide Over the Life Cycle* (eds S. J. Blumenthal & D. J. Kupfer), pp. 571–598. Washington, DC: APA.

GLOVER, G., MARKS, F. & NOWERS, M. (1989) Parasuicide in young Asian women. *British Journal of Psychiatry*, **154**, 271–272.

HANDY, S., CHITHIRAMOHAN, R., VALLARD, C., *et al* (1991) Ethnic differences in adolescent self-poisoning: a comparison of Asian and Caucasian groups. *Journal of Adolescence*, **14**, 157–162.

HAYNES, R. H. (1984) Suicide in Fiji: a preliminary study. *British Journal of Psychiatry*, **145**, 433–438.

—— (1987) Suicide and social response in Fiji: a historical survey. *British Journal of Psychiatry*, **151**, 21–26.

HEADLEY, L. (1981) Hong Kong. In *Suicide in Asia and the Near East* (ed. L. Headley), pp. 87–100. Berkeley, CA: University of California Press.

JACK, R. (1992) *Women and Attempted Suicide.* Hove: Lawrence Earlbaum Associates.

KESSLER, R. & MCRAE, J. (1983) Trends in the relationship between sex and attempted suicide. *Journal of Health and Social Behaviour,* **24**, 98–110.

KHAN, M. & REZA, H. (1998) Gender differences in non-fatal suicidal behaviour in Pakistan. *Suicidal & Life Threatening Behaviour,* **28**, 62–68.

KONATAXAKIS, V., MARKIDIS, M., VASLAMATZIS, G., *et al* (1988) Attempted suicide by jumping: clinical and social features. *Acta Psychiatrica Scandinavica,* **77**, 435–437.

LE VACHIA, C., LUCCHINI, F. & LEVI, F. (1994) Worldwide trends in suicide morality 1955–1989. *Acta Psychiatrica Scandinavica,* **90**, 53–64.

MCGIBBEN, L., BALLARD, C., HANDY, S., *et al* (1992) Deliberate self poisoning in Asian and Caucasian 12–15 year olds. *British Journal of Psychiatry,* **161**, 110–112.

MAHY, G. (1993) Suicide behaviour in the Caribbean. *International Review of Psychiatry,* **5**, 261–269.

MANIAM, T. (1988) Suicide and parasuicide in a hill resort in Malaysia. *British Journal of Psychiatry,* **153**, 222–225.

MAY, P. (1987) Suicide and self-destruction among American Indian youths. *American Indian and Alaska Native Mental Health Research,* **1**, 52–69.

MERRILL, J. & OWENS, J. (1986) Ethnic differences in self-poisoning – a comparison of Asian and White groups. *British Journal of Psychiatry,* **148**, 708–712.

—— & —— (1988) Self-poisoning among four immigrant groups. *Acta Psychiatrica Scandinavica,* **77**, 77–80.

NAGY, S. & ADCOCK, A. (1990) *The Alabama Adolescent Health Survey: Health Knowledge and Behaviours* , Report 11. Alabama: University of Alabama and Troy State University.

NATIONAL CENTER FOR HEALTH STATISTICS (1988) *Vital Statistics of the United States 1986,* Vol. 11, Publication PH588-1122. Washington, DC: Department of Health and Human Services.

NAZROO, J. (1997) *Ethnicity and Mental Health.* London: Policy Studies Institute.

NISSEN, T. & HAGGAG, A. (1988) Parasuicidal snow-wandering in Arctic Northern Norway. *Acta Psychiatric Scandinavica,* **77**, 309–313.

ODEJIDE, A. O., WILLIAMS, A. O., OHAERI, J. U., *et al* (1986) The epidemiology of deliberate self-harm: the Ibadam experience. *British Journal of Psychiatry,* **149**, 734–737.

PENG, K. & CHOO, A. (1986) Suicide and parasuicide in Singapore. *Medicine, Science and Law,* **30**, 225–233.

PLATT, S., BILLE-BRAHE, U., KERKHOF, A. *et al* (1992) Parasuicide in Europe: the WHO/EURO multi-centre study on parasuicide. Introduction and preliminary analysis for 1989. *Acta Psychiatrica Scandinavica,* **85**, 97–104.

PONNUDURAI, R., JEYAKAR, J. & SARASWALTRY, M. (1986) Attempted suicides in Madras. *Indian Journal of Psychiatry,* **28**, 59–62.

——, VIVEKANATHAN, V., RAJU, B., *et al* (1991) Attempted suicide: a two-year follow-up study. *Indian Journal of Psychiatry,* **33**, 291–292.

REE, G. (1971) Suicide in Macauta province, Fiji: a review of 73 cases. *The Practitioner,* **207**, 669–671.

RUBINSTEIN, J., HEERAN, T., HOUSEMAN, D., *et al* (1989) Suicidal behaviour in 'normal' adolescents: risk and protective factors. *Americal Journal of Orthopsychiatry,* **59**, 59–71.

SATHYAVATHI, K. (1971) Attempted suicide in psychiatric patients. *Indian Journal of Psychiatry,* **13**, 37–42.

SATO, T., TAKEICHI, M. & HARA, T. (1993) Suicide attempts by agricultural chemicals. *Indian Journal of Psychiatry,* **35**, 209–210.

TINKER, H. (1974) *A New System of Slavery: The Export of Indian Labour Overseas 1830–1920.* Oxford: Open University Press.

US DEPARTMENT OF HEALTH & HUMAN SERVICES (1985) *Report of the Secretary's Task Force on Black and Minority Health,* Vol. 1. Washington, DC: US Government Printing Office.

VAILLANT, G. & BLUMENTHAL, S. (1990) Introduction: suicide over the life cycle. In *Suicide Over the Life Cycle* (eds S. J. Blumenthal & D. J. Kupfer), pp. 1–16. Washington: APA.

VAN HOOFF, A. (1994) Suicide in antiquity. From kin killing to self-murder. In *Divergent Perspectives on Suicidal Behaviour* (ed. M. J. Kelleher), pp. 157–169. Cork: University of Cork.

VENKOBA RAO, A. (1965) Attempted suicide: an analysis of 114 medical admissions. *Indian Journal of Psychiatry*, **7**, 253.

—— (1981) India. In *Suicide in Asia and the Near East* (ed. L. Headley), pp. 210–228. Berkeley, CA: University of California Press.

—— & Chinnian, R. (1972) Attempted suicide and suicide in "students" in Madurai. *Indian Journal of Psychiatry*, **14**, 389.

WRIGHT, N., TRETHOWAN, W. N. & OWENS, J. (1981) Ethnic differences in self-poisoning. *Postgraduate Medical Journal*, **57**, 792–793.

YAP, P. (1958) *Suicide in Hong Kong.* Hong Kong: Hong Kong University Press.

13 Postnatal depression in Japanese women who have given birth in England

K. YOSHIDA, N. KIBE, M. N. MARKS, H. YAMASHITA, A. MATSUMOTO, H. NAKANO, N. TASHIRO and R. KUMAR

There are three main psychiatric disorders associated with childbirth. 'Maternity blues' are most common with an incidence of 50–80% in the UK and the USA (Yalom *et al*, 1968; Pitt, 1973; Stein, 1980; Kennerley & Gath, 1989; O'Hara *et al*, 1990; Hannah *et al*, 1992) (see Table 1). The blues are transient emotional disturbances, typically occurring around the fourth or fifth day after birth and usually lasting for a few hours or, at most, a day or two. The symptoms of the blues are generally recognised by the following: feeling low, crying, poor appetite, anxiety, headache, tenseness, poor concentration, restlessness, forgetfulness, irritability and confusion.

TABLE 1
Incidence of maternity blues

Authors	Country	Incidence (*n*)	%	Criterion
Yalom *et al* (1968)	USA	39	66	Tearfulness
Pitt (1973)	UK	100	50	Tearfulness or depression
Stein (1980)	UK	37	76	Tearfulness
Kennerley & Gath (1989)	UK	87	43	Kennerley scale
O'Hara *et al* (1990)	USA	182	42	Pitt scale
Hannah *et al* (1992)	LTK	42	50	Stein
Okano *et al* (1991)	Japan	325	26	Stein
Yoshida *et al* (1993)	Japan	160	13	Yalom
Yamashita *et al* (1995a)	Japan	378	34	Stein
Yoshida (1995)	Japanese in UK	100	37	Stein

Using these symptoms, Stein (1980) developed screening criteria for the blues. Characteristic psychological aspects of the blues were described by Kumar (1990):

> "By definition the blues are dysphoric reactions, although they may be intermingled with normal feelings of happiness and achievement which follow the birth".

Sometimes the symptoms are so severe and persistent that the situation may be that of a developing clinical depression. There are no definite conclusions about correlations between the blues and obstetric complications or breast-feeding (Pitt, 1973; Stein, 1980; Nott *et al*, 1976; Cox *et al*, 1982; Hapgood *et al*, 1988; Kendell *et al*, 1981), environmental stress (Pitt, 1973; Kennerley & Gath, 1989) or personality (Harris, 1980; Kennerley & Gath, 1989; Kumar & Robson, 1984).

Postnatal depression is experienced by 10–15% of mothers in the UK and the USA (Pitt, 1968; Wolkind *et al*, 1980; Playfair & Gowers, 1981; Cox *et al*, 1982; Kumar & Robson, 1984; Watson *et al*, 1984; Cooper *et al*, 1988; O'Hara *et al*, 1990; Cox *et al*, 1993; see Table 2).

The clinical manifestations of postnatal depression are the same as those of depression in other settings. The onset is within the first two or three months after giving birth. General practitioners (GPs) usually treat women suffering from postnatal depression at their clinics. However, if the symptoms are severe, they refer mothers to psychiatrists for more specialist treatment (Kumar *et al*, 1995).

The main aetiological factors of postnatal depression are psycho-social. Problems in early parental relationships, problems in current marital and family relationships, lack of social support, a past history of depression, ambivalence about the pregnancy, and social and obstetric stress are the most commonly found concomitants (Paykel *et al*, 1980; O'Hara *et al*, 1983, 1984; Kumar & Robson, 1984, Kumar, 1990; Marks *et al*, 1992).

Puerperal psychosis is very rare and occurs in one out of every 1000 live births. The onset is usually within two weeks after delivery (Meltzer & Kumar, 1985; Kendell *et al*, 1987) with symptoms such as confusion or stuporous states, delusions, hallucinations, and manic or depressive mood disturbance.

Post-partum psychosis is thought to have a greater biological component than postnatal depression, whereas the latter is more environmentally or culturally based. The incidence of severe mental illness following childbirth in Europe and America appears to be independent of social, cultural, educational, nutritional and medical developments. In addition, incidence rates reported in Tanzania, Saudi Arabia and Japan are the within the range reported in

TABLE 2
Incidence of postnatal depression

Authors	Country	n	Time of interview	Incidence (%)	Classification system
Pitt (1968)	UK	305	6–8 weeks	10.8	Questionnaire and clinical interviews
Wolkind *et al* (1980)	UK	117	4 months	10.0	PSE
Playfair & Gowers (1981)	UK	618	3 months	10.0	Symptoms and checklist
Cox *et al* (1982)	UK	105	4 months	13.0	CIS
Kumar & Robson (1984)	UK	119	3 months	13.9	CIS and RDC
Watson *et al* (1984)	UK	128	6 weeks	12.0	CIS and ICD–9
Cooper *et al* (1988)	UK	460	3 months	8.7	PSE
O'Hara *et al* (1990)	USA	182	9 weeks	10.4	RDC
Cox *et al* (1993)	UK	232	5 weeks	7.0	RDC
Aoki *et al* (1989)	Japan	120	1 months	9.3	RDC
Okano & Nomura (1992)	Japan	47	1 month	8.5	RDC
Yamashita *et al* (1995*b*)	Japan	72	3 months	13.9	RDC
Yoshida (1995)	Japanese in UK	88	3 months	12.5	RDC

CIS, Clinical Interview Schedule; PSE, Present State Examination; EPDS, Edinburgh Postnatal Depression Scale; RDC, Research Diagnostic Criteria.

developed nations (Kumar, 1994). Kumar (1994) suggested that some factors unique to the reproductive process may be predominantly responsible for the puerperal psychoses.

Significance of cross-cultural studies on mental illness associated with childbirth

Mental illness associated with childbirth provides a very useful way of investigating cultural differences, because social concepts about parenthood and traditional ways of having a baby vary in different cultures or countries, whereas the biological mechanisms involved will be constant across cultures. Kumar (1994) suggests that:

> "The trans-cultural approach to postnatal psychiatric disorders provides a unique opportunity not only to test hypotheses about social and cultural contributions to the etiology of psychotic and

non psychotic reactions to childbirth, but also an opportunity to study the ways in which social factors can influence the evolution of psychopathology."

Cultural aspects of childbirth in Japan

Traditionally, at around 32–35 weeks' gestation, most Japanese women return to their own family homes to give birth and remain there with their babies and other older children, if they have any, receiving emotional and practical support from their families, particularly their mothers. About two months after delivery, they return to their marital homes to join their husbands. Nowadays, Japanese daily life has become more Westernised. However, this tradition, which is called *satogaeribunben (satogaeri* means returning to wives' parents' homes, *bunben* means delivery), is still not uncommon. If it is not possible for pregnant women to undertake *satogaeribunben*, grandmothers instead go to their daughters' marital homes to look after them and their babies. A recent survey of *satogaeribunben* was reported by Yamashita *et al* (1995*a*), who found that 174 out of 270 pregnant women (64.4%) delivered their baby by *satogaeribunben*. Rates of *satogaeribunben* vary in different cities, towns and villages.

There are some disadvantages to this traditional Japanese system in terms of obstetric and paediatric concerns. Almost all Japanese women deliver their babies in hospital. If they return to their home town to give birth, pregnancy monitoring is disrupted, in that there is a necessary medical handover between midwives or obstetricians from a woman's marital home town to her family's home town. There may also be deleterious effects on the new infant, for example the move back to the marital home usually takes place at a time when the infant's immunoglobulin G level is likely to be low. In addition the long period of marital separation means that fathers are excluded from not only their wives but also their children, and this can create psychological problems in family members. Regardless of these possible adverse aspects, this tradition has been regarded as a great support system for women giving birth.

Maternity blues and postnatal depression in Japanese mothers in Japan

Japanese mothers studied in Japan appear to show a lower incidence of the blues than Western mothers. The incidence of the blues reported by Yoshida *et al* (1993) using Yalom's criteria (Yalom *et al*, 1968) was 13%. Using Stein's criteria for the blues, Okano *et al* (1991) and Yamashita *et al* (1995a) reported incidences of 26% and 34%, respectively. These are much lower than rates in the UK and USA.

In contrast to the blues, Japanese mothers in Japan show nearly the same incidence of postnatal depression when measured using standard Western diagnostic interviews such as the Schedule for Affective Disorders and Schizophrenia (SADS; Spitzer & Endicott, 1978a). However, when depression is measured by self-report, for example using the Edinburgh Postnatal Depression Scale (EPDS; Cox *et al*, 1987), they tend to score lower than Western women. Studies in which clinical diagnosis was made by diagnostic interview using the SADS as well as the EPDS have shown that a lower EPDS cut-off point of nine, instead of the UK cut-off of 13, is a better predictor for probable postnatal depression (Okano *et al*, 1996). There are, of course, problems of category fallacy (see Chapter 11).

The lower incidences of the blues and postnatal depression in Japanese women, using Stein's blues scales and the EPDS, respectively, support the view that Japanese women may be less likely to express negative feelings in self-report questionnaires than Western women, that is, that Western self-report instruments are less sensitive to moderate mood disturbances in Japanese women. It seems that only in probing, face-to-face interviews with a skilled interviewer are symptoms properly elucidated.

Another possible explanation, especially for the lower incidence of the blues in Japan, is that Japanese mothers receive more family and social support (e.g. *satogaeribunben*) throughout the perinatal period. Grandmothers help the new mothers with domestic work at home and this enables the new mothers to have physical rest especially during the very early postnatal days when the blues usually occur. Also, the new mothers may have practical and psychological support from the grandmothers in terms of baby care. However, this support might not be so effective as to prevent the onset of postnatal depression, especially when it occurs around the timing of withdrawal of a grandmother's support.

One way of testing the relative contribution of family support is to investigate Japanese women living in England and compare them with perinatal Japanese women living in Japan. Women separated from their own culture might show higher rates of the blues or postnatal depression than women in Japan. Further, does the presence of the grandmother who comes to the UK to look after her daughter and baby reduce the incidence of the blues or postnatal depression?

Delivering babies abroad: pregnant and postnatal Japanese women in the UK

Japanese people living in the UK

In 1993, 39 071 Japanese people lived in Greater London. In 1994, 29 146 Japanese people lived in Greater London (data were obtained from the Japanese Embassy, 1995). More than half were Japanese businessmen and their families and 30% were researchers or young students. Japanese businessmen usually stay in the UK for 3–6 years with their wives and children. More than 400 Japanese mothers give birth in the UK each year. In 1994, 495 babies were registered with the Japanese Embassy. Compared with other ethnic minority groups, only a small proportion of the Japanese people in the UK are permanent residents (see Table 3).

Japanese women living in the UK and *Nakayoshi-Kai*

Living abroad can be stressful and having a baby abroad has particular difficulties. There is a language barrier, especially between the mother and the midwives and obstetricians. Living in a different country also makes it much more difficult to obtain support from the extended family.

Nakayoshi-Kai (known as the Japanese Friendship Group) is a registered charity group supporting Japanese mothers and their families while they stay in Britain. It was set up in 1990, to address problems of loneliness and isolation among Japanese families living in UK. The group now has a membership of over 250 families (10% of which are mixed-marriage families) in the UK and Japan (for the few members who used to live in the UK and have now returned to Japan). All activities are voluntarily organised by members. These include publishing a bilingual

Table 3
Number of Japanese people living in the UK (data from Japanese Embassy, 1995)

Occupation	1993	(%)	1994	(%)
Businessman (company)	32 528	(57.7)	20 020	(43.9)
Researcher, student	17 333	(30.8)	18 601	(40.8)
Civil servant (government)	757	(1.3)	636	(1.4)
Others	2351	(4.2)	2379	(5.2)
Permanent resident	3386	(6.0)	3981	(8.7)
Total	56 335	(100.0)	45 617	(100.0)

Japanese/English newsletter, an 'open house' once a month in north and south London where Japanese mothers can meet new friends over tea or exchange information on raising children and the 'New Mums' meeting which supports mothers-to-be and mothers with babies of 18 months or younger. This meeting is supported by an English health visitor and *Nakayoshi-Kai* member to help Japanese mothers attend their local health clinic with a translation service. There is also a *Nakayoshi* library which contains 150 Japanese books on maternity and children for mothers, as well as 330 children's books in Japanese, and holds a story-telling time and other activities related to Japanese language and culture. There is also a telephone service which offers a wide range of Japanese specialists such as clinical psychologists, a gynaecologist, a psychiatrist, a midwife and other nurses and a dentist who are available to offer advice to Japanese mothers over the telephone.

Maternity pack

Nakayoshi-Kai has published a bilingual Japanese–English maternity information pack which contains a wide range of basic information about pregnancy and childbirth in the UK. Topics covered include details about registration for National Insurance, registration with a GP, contraception/abortion, an English–Japanese pregnancy word list, antenatal classes, a maternity shopping list, what to do when labour starts, phrases to use in a maternity ward around childbirth, emergency action/midwives' green cars, postnatal care and community midwives, health visitors, differences in immunisation systems between Japan and the UK, registering the birth and social security benefits and useful addresses for Japanese mothers such as Japanese clinics and chemists.

Mental health of Japanese women living in England in association with childbirth

We aimed to survey the incidence and some of the characteristic aspects of the maternity blues and, more importantly, postnatal depression among Japanese mothers living mainly in London and to compare these with Japanese mothers in Japan using the same methodology (Yoshida, 1995).

Subjects were recruited by a Japanese psychiatrist (K.Y.) from an antenatal class for pregnant Japanese women and their husbands in London or from an advertisement placed in the Japanese maternity pack discussed above. One hundred and twenty-two pregnant women agreed to take part in the study.

TABLE 4
*Prevalence of probable postnatal depression in Japanese women
screened by the Edinburgh Postnatal Depression Scale*

Authors	Country	n	Time of interview	Incidence (%)	Cut-off point
Okano *et al* (1991)	Japan	325	1 month	3.1	13
Okano *et al* (1995)	Japan	2531	4 months	11.7	9
Yamashita *et al* (1995*b*)	Japan	72	3 months	12.5	9
Yoshida (1995)	Japanese in the UK	88	3 months	8	9

The study was longitudinal, gathering information at four different time periods: late pregnancy and five days, one month and three months postnatally. The mothers completed several questionnaires and screening scales for maternity blues and postnatal depression.

At three months postnatally, the mothers were visited at home and interviewed using the SADS. This gave us the opportunity of finding out mothers' feelings more directly.

Thirty-seven per cent (*n*=100) of mothers who completed Stein's (1980) blues scale were categorised as having maternity blues (a score of eight or above). This incidence is less than is generally observed in the West, but higher than the incidence in Japan (see Table 1).

Twelve (12%) of 98 mothers who had been interviewed at three months post-partum were diagnosed as having had minor or major depressive disorder in the first three months. This is very similar to rates reported for Western mothers and nearly the same or slightly higher than in Japan (see Table 2). The peak onset of postnatal depression was one month after the delivery.

Seventy-six per cent of the grandmothers came to the UK to help the new mothers despite the long, expensive journey from Japan. However, the grandmothers' visit to the UK to help their daughters and grandchildren did not affect the occurrence of either maternity blues or postnatal depression.

Discussion

Incidence of maternity blues

The incidence of the blues varies in different studies even among Western women, as shown in Table 1. This is because different methods have been used to survey the presence of the blues.

Okano has produced a Japanese version of the Stein scales, using the double translation method, from English into Japanese and back to English. Yoshida in England and Yamashita in Japan used this Japanese version to survey the incidence of the blues. The data shown in Table 1 suggest that there is a lower incidence of the blues in Japanese mothers irrespective of where they live. This might be a reflection of the reputed stoicism of the Japanese character and the reluctance to show emotion, since in our study grandmothers' help did not make a difference in terms of the occurrence of the blues. It might still be possible that there is a positive aspect of grandmothers' support which makes the incidence of the blues lower in Japanese women, because, unlike postnatal depression, there is no diagnostic criteria of the blues based on observed symptoms by interviews. The incidences of the blues reported have been based only on self-report questionnaires.

Incidence of postnatal depression

Almost all the research on postnatal depression has been carried out in North America and Western European countries. There have been some Japanese studies and these are summarised in Table 2. Okano & Nomura (1992) studied 47 Japanese mothers at one month post-partum using the SADS interview and found that 8.5% of them were Research Diagnostic Criteria (RDC; Spitzer *et al*, 1978*b*) cases of depression.

Yamashita *et al* (1995*b*) reported a study of 72 Japanese mothers who were interviewed using SADS at three months postnatally; 13.9% were found to have had major or minor depressive disorder since delivery. In our study of postnatal depression in Japanese women in England, using the same method as Yamashita *et al* (1995*b*), the three-month postnatal prevalence was 12.5%. Thus, the prevalence of postnatal depression during the three months following childbirth, in Japanese women who have their babies in England, was very similar to that seen in Japanese women who had their babies in Japan, and also to rates found in studies of women in the UK and USA.

The EPDS (Cox *et al*, 1987), is a well-known screening question-naire for postnatal depression. It has 10 itemised questions which ask about moods and feelings, but excludes physical complaints, such as general fatigue and headaches, which are related to the general effects of childbearing.

Okano *et al* (1991) found that only 3.1% of subjects in his study scored 13 or more, which is the cut-off point used in the UK studies to detect probable postnatal depression. In our study there were 11

Japanese women with postnatal depression. However, none of these women scored 13 or higher on the EPDS. These results suggest that the EPDS is not sufficiently sensitive to detect postnatal depression in Japanese mothers when a cut-off point as high as that used in Western settings is applied. As Okano *et al* (1995) have also reported, when a cut-off point of nine was used, the prevalence of probable postnatal depression was similar to that detected using SADS interviews (see Table 4).

This difference in self-reporting of depressive symptoms may reflect a cultural difference in the women's willingness to talk about their feelings. However, when the women were asked by a psychiatrist within a structured interview, evidence about their mood state became available. The EPDS questionnaire focuses only on mood and emotion and excludes physical symptoms. Japanese women tend to express emotional complaints by referring to physical problems or worries about child care rather than by expressing their feelings when they are depressed (also see Chapter 5). Upadhyaya *et al* (1989) have also reported that Asian women in the UK who had psychiatric symptoms and attended a well-baby clinic consulted a doctor predominantly for somatic symptoms.

Most Japanese women with postnatal depression in England developed their symptoms around one month postnatally. The reason for this seems to be that fatigue due to delivery and child care reaches a peak at this time and it was also at this time that the grandmothers returned to Japan. Not only women who suffered from postnatal depression, but also women who remained well, confessed that they were anxious and tense about the withdrawal of their mothers' support. Yamashita *et al* (1995*b*) and Okano *et al* (1991) also found the same time of onset in Japanese women in Japan – Okano *et al* (1991) have also suggested that discontinuation of grandmothers' help when *satogaeribunben* periods were over may be a precipitating factor.

Prodromal symptoms of postnatal depression

Having severe or prolonged blues or excessive worry about baby care can be risk factors for postnatal depression. Several studies have reported a correlation between the blues and postnatal depression (Pitt, 1968; Playfair & Gowers, 1981; Cox *et al*, 1982; Hapgood *et al*, 1988; Hannah *et al*, 1992). Most of the Japanese women in our study who became depressed had earlier been categorised as having maternity blues. Their chief complaints were physical problems and worries about baby care such as poor weight gain, breast-feeding and the baby's crying.

Conclusions

In Japan the average number of children per married couple has been decreasing year by year and recently it has been below 1.5. Consequently mothers now tend to pay more attention to quality of child care such as the emotional development of their babies and mother–infant bonding. However, mothers still tend to sacrifice themselves, hiding their own emotional problems and trying not to disturb their husbands' daily life and work. Japanese women are socially expected to view their roles as mothers as more important than their roles as wives. Their personal identity is seen as least important. Members of the obstetric staff realise that dealing with delivery in a mechanical way is no longer appropriate and pay more attention to women's mental care. This means that they usually consult psychiatrists about their 'patient mothers' who are apparently either severely depressed or psychotic, but they still need to be more aware of women with minor depressive symptoms.

What is needed is careful monitoring, especially of Japanese women who experience maternity blues or complain about physical problems even in the absence of emotional problems in the early puerperal period, and also education about mental state in association with childbirth for normal pregnant and postnatal women. To this end, a flexible liaison arrangement between obstetric staff and psychiatrists or psychologists would seem to be important.

Acknowledgements

The survey of the postnatal mental state of Japanese women both in Japan (Yamashita *et al*, 1995*a,b*; Okano *et al*, 1995) and England (Yoshida, 1995) was supported by a grant from the Japanese Ministry of Health and Welfare from 1993 to 1995. (The chief grant holder was H.N.)

References

AOKI, M., KITAMURA, T., SINIA, S., *et al* (1989) Baby blues project (in Japanese). In *Hattatsu (Development)*, Vol. 9 (eds K. Okonogi & H. Waranabe), pp. 74–79. Tokyo: Atnerva shobou.
COOPER, P. J., CAMPBELL, E. A, DAY, A., *et al* (1988) Non-psychotic disorder after childbirth: a prospective study of prevalence, incidence, course and nature. *British Journal of Psychiatry*, **152**, 799–806.
COX, J. L., CONNOR, Y. & KENDELL, R. E. (1982) Prospective study of the psychiatric disorders of childbirth. *British Journal of Psychiatry*, **140**, 111–117.
——, HOLDEN, M. & SAGOVSKY, R. (1987) Detection of postnatal depression: Development of the 10-item Edinburgh Postnatal Depression Scale. *British Journal of Psychiatry*, **150**, 782–786.

——, MURAY, D. & CHAPMAN, G. (1993) A controlled study of the onset, duration and prevalence of postnatal depression. *British Journal of Psychiatry*, **163**, 27–31.

HANNAH, P., ADAMS, D., LEE, A., *et al* (1992) Links between early post-partum mood and postnatal depression. *British Journal of Psychiatry*, **160**, 777–780.

HAPGOOD, C. C., ELKIND, G. S. & WRIGHT, J. J. (1988) Maternity blues: Phenomena and relationship to later post-partum depression. *Australian & New Zealand Journal of Psychiatry*, **22**, 299–306.

HARRIS, B. (1980) Prospective trial of L-tryptophan in maternity blues. *British Journal of Psychiatry*, **137**, 233–235.

KENDELL, R. E., MCGUIRE, R. J., CONNOR, Y., *et al* (1981) Mood changes in the first weeks after childbirth. *Journal of Affective Disorders*, **3**, 317–326.

——, CHAHNERS, J. C. & PLATZ, C. (1987) Epidemiology of puerperal psychoses. *British Journal of Psychiatry*, **150**, 662–673.

KENNERLEY, H. & GATH, D. (1989) Maternity blues. 1. Detection and measurement by questionnaire. *British Journal of Psychiatry*, **155**, 356–362.

KUMAR, R. (1990) Childbirth and mental health. *Triangle*, **29**, 73–81.

—— (1994) Postnatal mental illness: a transcultural perspective. *Social Psychiatry and Psychiatric Epidemiology*, **29**, 250–264.

—— & ROBSON, K. M. (1984) A prospective study of emotional disorders in childbearing women. *British Journal of Psychiatry*, **144**, 35–47.

——, MARKS, M. N., PLATZ, C., *et al* (1995) Clinical survey of a psychiatric mother and baby unit: characteristics of 100 consecutive admissions. *Journal of Affective Disorders*, **33**, 11–22.

MARKS, M. N., WIECK, A., CHECKLEY, S. A., *et al* (1992) Contribution of psychological and social factors to psychotic and non-psychotic relapse after childbirth in women with histories of affective disorder. *Journal of Affective Disorders*, **29**, 253–264.

MELTZER, E. S. & KUMAR, R. (1985) Puerperal mental illness, clinical features and classification: a study of 142 mother and baby admissions. *British Journal of Psychiatry*, **147**, 647–654.

NOTT, P. N., FRANKLIN, M., ARMITAGE, C., *et al* (1976) Hormonal changes and mood in the puerperium. *British Journal of Psychiatry*, **128**, 379–383.

O'HARA, M. W., REHM, L. P. & CAMPBELL, S. B. (1983) Postpartum depression: a role for social network and life stress variables. *Journal of Nervous Mental Disorders*, **171**, 336–341.

OKANO, T., NEUNABER, D. J. & ZEROSKI, E. M. (1984) A prospective study of postpartum depression: prevalence, course and predictive factors. *Journal of Abnormal Psychology*, **93**, 158–171.

——, ZEKOSKI, E. M., PHILLIPS, L. R. *et al* (1990) Controlled prospective study of postpartum mood disorders: comparison of childbearing and non-childbearing women. *Journal of Abnormal Psychology*, **99**, 3–15.

———, NOMURA, J., KOSHIKAWA, N., *et al* (1991) Cross-cultural study of maternity blues and postpartum depression (in Japanese with an English abstract). *Japanese Journal of Clinical Psychiatry*, **33**, 1051–1058.

—— & NOMURA, J. (1992) Endocrine study of the maternity blues. *Progress in Neuro-Psychopharmacology & Biological Psychiatry*, **16**, 921–932.

——, TAMAKI, R., MASUCHI, F., *et al* (1995) Epidemiological study on incidences of postpartum mental disorders in the Japanese women in Mie prefecture (in Japanese with an English abstract). In *Biological and Psycho-Social Factors During Pregnancy and the Postpartum Period and the Physical and Mental Health of Mothers and Infants* (ed. H. Nakano), pp. 31–36. Tokyo: Japanese Government Ministry of Health and Welfare.

———, MARURA, M., MASUJI, F., *et al* (1996) Validation and reliability of a Japanese version of the EPDS. *Archives of Psychiatric Diagnosis and Clinical Evaluation*, **7**, 525–533.

PAYKEL, E. S., EMMS, E. M., FLETCHER, J., *et al* (1980) Life events and social support in puerperal depression. *British Journal of Psychiatry*, **136**, 339–346.

PITT, B. (1968) Atypical depression following childbirth. *British Journal of Psychiatry*, **114**, 1325–1335.

—— (1973) Maternity blues. *British Journal of Psychiatry*, **122**, 431–433.

PLAYFAIR, H. R. & GOWERS, J. I. (1981) Depression following childbirth – a search for predictive signs. *Journal of the Royal College of General Practitioners*, **31**, 201–208.

SPITZER, R. L. & ENDICOTT, J. (1978*a*) *Schedule for the Affective Disorders and Schizophrenia (SADS)* (3rd edn). New York: Biometrics Research Department, New York State Psychiatric Institute.

——, ENDICOTT, J. & ROBINS, E. (1978*b*) *Research Diagnostic Criteria (RDC) for a Selected Group of Functional Disorders* (3rd edn). New York: Biometrics Research Department, New York State Psychiatric Institute.

STEIN, G. (1980) The pattern of mental change and body weight change in the first postpartum week. *Journal of Psychosomatic Research*, **24**, 165–171.

UPADHYAYA, A., CREED, F. & UPADHYAYA, M. (1989) Psychiatric morbidity among mothers attending well-baby clinic: a cross-cultural comparison. *Acta Psychiatrica Scandinavica*, **81**, 148–151.

WATSON, J. P., ELLIOT, S. A., RUGG, A. J., *et al* (1984) Psychiatric disorder in pregnancy and the first postnatal year. *British Journal of Psychiatry*, **144**, 453–462.

WOLKIND, S., ZAJICEK, E. & GHODSIAN, M. (1980) Continuities in maternal depression. *International Journal of Family Psychiatry*, **1**, 167–182.

YALOM, I. D., LUNDE, D. T., MOOS, R. H., *et al* (1968) Postpartum blues syndrome. *Archives of General Psychiatry*, **18**, 16–27.

YAMASHITA, H., ASOU, T., OKANO, T. *et al* (1995*a*) Multi-centre prospective study of early postpartum mood in Japanese women (in Japanese). In *Biological and Psycho-Social Factors During Pregnancy and the Postpartum Period and the Physical and Mental Health of Mothers and Infants* (ed. H. Nakano), pp. 165–167. Tokyo: Japanese Government Ministry of Health and Welfare.

——, GOTO, E., NAKANE, H., *et al* (1995*b*) The longitudinal survey of the incidence of maternity blues and postnatal depression: The use of modified Western screening tests and intervention for the Japanese (in Japanese with an English abstract). In *Biological and Psycho-Social Factors During Pregnancy and the Postpartum Period and the Physical and Mental Health of Mothers and Infants* (ed. H. Nakano), pp. 26–30. Tokyo: Japanese Government Ministry of Health and Welfare.

—— (1995) Postnatal mental health of the Japanese women who have given birth in England (in Japanese with an English abstract). In *Biological and Psycho-Social Factors During Pregnancy and the Postpartum Period and the Physical and Mental Health of Mothers and Infants* (ed. H. Nakano), pp. 37–39. Tokyo: Japanese Government Ministry of Health and Welfare.

——, KUMAR, R., MATSUMOTO, A., *et al* (1993) Maternity blues and postnatal depression in Japan. *Marce Bulletin*, Spring, 15–18.

14 Forensic psychiatry

TONY MADEN

Forensic psychiatry deals primarily with mentally disordered offenders. The definition is sometimes broadened to include 'those who show similar behaviours' in recognition of the fact that many offences committed by people with mental disorders do not lead to prosecutions because of the obvious presence of mental illness. It is a very specialised area, as the overlap between criminality and psychiatric disorder is small in numerical terms. Few psychiatric patients are offenders, and most offenders do not have a psychiatric disorder. Despite the relatively small number of patients involved, forensic psychiatry has a high profile. It is subject to frequent critical scrutiny, because it is mainly concerned with compulsory treatment and because serious offences by people with mental disorders receive excessive media attention.

Concern is often expressed regarding the ethnicity of psychiatric patients receiving compulsory treatment. People of African–Caribbean descent are over-represented in both offender and patient populations, relative to their proportion in the community at large. The prevalence of psychiatric disorder in ethnic minorities is discussed in other chapters (4, 5 and 6) but, before considering forensic psychiatry in more detail, it is necessary to deal briefly with the relationship between ethnicity and offending.

Ethnicity and offending

People of African–Caribbean origin make up about 5% of the general population of England and Wales, but they account for 11% of men and 25% of women in the sentenced prison population (Home Office, 1993). The figure for women is misleading, as it is inflated by the presence of a large number of women imprisoned for drug smuggling, who are normally resident in West Africa (Maden et al, 1992). However, the figures carry a clear message – as noted in Chapter

2, there are approximately twice as many people of African–Caribbean origin in the sentenced prison population as would be expected if prisoners were drawn at random from the general population. Of course, prisoners are not drawn at random from the general population. Although discrimination by the courts may play a role (Hood, 1992), the over-representation of certain ethnic groups in prison reflects differential rates of offending. The statistics are often misused by politicians, particularly by those with eugenic tendencies, but they cannot be explained in terms of genetic differences, and should be seen as an example of cultural and economic influences on offending (Maden, 1993). Ethnic minority groups are not evenly distributed across the country, but are concentrated in certain geographical areas and socio-economic groups. People from ethnic minority groups are more likely to live in areas that have suffered disproportionately from the decline of the manufacturing industry and that have high rates of poverty and unemployment. Therefore, the association between ethnic origin and offending may be an artefact resulting from social and economic factors which have a statistical association with both offending and ethnic origin.

This explanation is a criminological or sociological one, which deals with crime as if it were a simple variable for scientific measurement and analysis. In addition, the political dimension must not be forgotten. Crime is socially defined. It is not a single variable, and it is unlikely that any one mechanism will explain all offending. In the USA and South Africa Black people achieved full civil rights only because many people were prepared to break the law, risking penalties which included death. These struggles are a part of recent, living memory, in a way which the past struggles of White people are not. It is inevitable that they inform current attitudes to the law, especially where economic injustices persist, and some British police forces make regular out-of-court settlements to deal with allegations of racist behaviour on the part of their officers. These matters may seem far removed from disputes over the use of cannabis in secure psychiatric units, but they are necessary for a full understanding of the attitudes involved.

In many parts of England and Wales, services for offenders spend much of their time dealing with members of ethnic minorities. They cannot function properly without an awareness of the cultural dimensions of their work. This is also true of secure psychiatric units, where the picture is complicated by mental illness and compulsory detention.

Ethnic composition of secure hospital populations

A national survey of admissions to secure units in England and Wales found that 20% of patients were of African–Caribbean origin (Jones &

Berry, 1986). In a more recent survey of admissions to a medium secure unit in the West Midlands, the figure was 38% (Cope & Ndegwa, 1990). In a medium secure unit serving parts of south London, it is usual for a majority of patients to be of African–Caribbean origin.

The reasons for the preponderance of African–Caribbean patients in medium secure facilities are not known. As in the case of all offending, it seems likely that it is partly a result of a higher prevalence of mentally disordered offending. It is possible that discrimination makes a contribution, but this requires the assumption that White mentally disordered offenders are not admitted to medium secure units, even when their clinical presentation is similar to that of Black patients who are admitted. There is no evidence to support this proposition as a general explanation. Patients in medium secure units have usually committed serious offences that would have resulted in imprisonment, had they not been hospitalised. Among sentenced prisoners, there is evidence to suggest that serious mental illness is more common among people of African–Caribbean origin, where the prevalence has been measured at 6%, compared with 2% in White prisoners (Maden, 1995). Far from suggesting that White patients are less likely to receive compulsory treatment after committing an offence, a more feasible interpretation of these figures is that discrimination sometimes works to prevent Black mentally disordered offenders from receiving the treatment they need, in hospital, resulting in them being sent to prison instead.

It is also significant that members of ethnic minorities are under-represented among patients detained under the Mental Health Act 1983 category of psychopathic disorder. The diagnosis of personality disorder is notoriously unreliable, so any general tendency to 'psychiatrise' ethnic minority offending would be expected to result in a higher proportion of Black patients in this category. Instead, it may be evidence of a tendency to be more punitive towards ethnic minority offenders, with doctors and the courts choosing punishment rather than treatment. The evidence from sentenced prisoners does not support this suggestion. There does not appear to be a large pool of unidentified personality disorder within ethnic minority prisoners, where rates of this diagnosis are lower than in White prisoners. Of course, there may be under-diagnosis of personality disorder in Black inmates, but the 'hard' data which are available do not support this explanation. For example, the prevalence rates of deliberate self-harm, injecting drugs and alcohol misuse (behaviours which frequently accompany personality disorder) are all lower in prisoners from ethnic minorities. Although further research is needed into this complex question, it is not surprising that the prevalence of personality disorder should vary in different cultural groups. The reasons are speculative, but may include cultural differences in child-rearing practices.

There may be doubt about the reasons for the lack of Black patients detained because of personality disorder, but one consequence is clear: the statistics on ethnic origin understate the ethnic differences in patients detained because of mental illness (because almost all Black patients in secure units have this diagnosis, whereas a significant proportion of White patients are detained because of personality disorder). It follows that the single most important factor in achieving a reduction in the proportion of Black patients would be the develop-ment of more effective ways of managing schizophrenia.

Implications for practice

Although the reasons for the excess of Black patients in medium secure units are not fully understood it is possible to consider some of the implications of their presence. Within some services, Black patients form a clear majority. Therefore, they suffer disproportionately from any problems which affect the service as a whole. In the case of medium secure facilities, the most pressing of these problems is a national shortage of beds. Although the Butler Committee (Home Office & Department of Health and Social Security, 1975) suggested in 1975 that about 2000 beds would be needed nationally, there were only 800 National Health Service medium secure beds in operation more than 20 years later. As a consequence, patients are often sent to private hospitals. Most of these patients come from cities (usually London), however, most of the hospitals are located in distant parts of the country, including North Yorkshire, North Wales and Cambridgeshire. Patients may be treated hundreds of miles away from their families, and away from the environment with which they are familiar. The location of the units is often rural, as this reduces costs. It may therefore be difficult to recruit staff from ethnic minorities, and White staff may have had little contact with members of ethnic minorities, or with inner-city life, except in the course of their work. A recent inquiry into a homicide by a psychiatric patient criticised his care at Kneesworth House, saying that it was "barely adequate" to his needs and appeared solely custodial. The inquiry team also criticised the fact that there was inadequate sensitivity to the needs of Black patients at the hospital (East London and the City Health Authority, 1995). The rehabilitation of patients held far from their homes may also be complicated. It is difficult to maintain close links between the in-patient team and those who will provide out-patient care and supervision. Close working relationships lead to the development of mutual trust, and the absence of such trust is likely to lead to patients spending longer in secure conditions, as local teams will be wary of taking over their care.

The shortage of medium secure beds also has consequences in other parts of the system. Prisoners have to wait longer for transfer to hospital, after their mental disorder has been diagnosed. Adequate treatment is delayed, and there is a significant risk of suicide. At the other extreme, there are long delays for patients waiting to move from maximum security special hospitals as part of their rehabilitation.

So far, it has been argued that Black patients form a majority, or a substantial minority, in many forensic psychiatric settings, so their interests coincide with those of patients as a whole. It would be misleading to pretend that there are no special factors to be considered. The issue of racial discrimination means that staff recruitment and training need particular care. A difficult balance must be maintained. Patients in many forensic settings have serious restrictions on their liberty, which were usually imposed by a court but must be enforced by hospital staff. Many patients, whether Black or White, lack any insight into their illness, and believe that they have been wrongly detained. In these circumstances, it is easy for a patient's resentment to become channelled along ethnic lines. At the same time, there may be insensitivity on the part of the hospital to ethnic issues. The challenge for staff is to restrict a patient's freedom only to the extent necessitated by the risk of harm to themselves or others, while respecting the patient's right to be different in other ways.

This problem is particularly difficult for those parts of forensic psychiatry which still provide long-term in-patient care, now obsolete in many other branches of psychiatry. The average stay for a patient in a special hospital is about eight years, and the length of stay in medium secure units is increasing, so that many patients will now exceed the intended maximum of about two years. Long-term medium secure units are being developed, some of which will provide for indefinite admissions.

Long-stay units soon fall prey to institutionalisation, of both staff and patients. Patients can find their freedom restricted in a variety of ways, not because of any threat to safety, but simply because of the traditions developed on a ward over a number of years. When staff and patients tend to come from different ethnic groups, such problems can easily lead to the unthinking suppression of a patient's cultural identity. Greater recruitment of staff from ethnic minority groups is an important part of the response to these problems (see Chapter 22), but it is an over-simplification to see the problem only in these terms. Even when staff and patients are drawn from the same ethnic groups, there are likely to be many differences in terms of educational background, social class and life experience. A greater sensitivity to the needs of the offender/patient cannot be assumed. Furthermore, attempts to match staff and patients can soon become absurd: should staff include a certain proportion of ex-prisoners, or people with serious mental illness? Instead, there is a need for active strategies to combat the effects of institutionalisation, mainly by continuing staff training and maintaining good supervision.

Cannabis and secure psychiatric facilities

Many secure psychiatric units spend a disproportionate amount of time policing the attempts of patients to use cannabis. The known facts about cannabis are that it can cause toxic, psychotic reactions if taken in large doses, although there is doubt as to whether it can cause a persistent psychosis, in the manner of amphetamines (see Chapter 6). Of greater importance to the present discussion, it is also known to cause relapse, or a worsening of symptoms, in those who suffer from a schizophrenic or affective psychosis. The effects vary between patients in unpredictable ways. Some appear sensitive to small doses of the drug and others appear to be unaffected by large amounts. Neuroleptic medication may protect some patients from the effects of cannabis, while having no such effect in others.

There are frequent confrontations between staff and patients. Patients can always find an example of someone who appears unaffected by cannabis and staff can point out the opposite. The issue soon becomes an ethnic one, as cannabis is given particular significance by the Rastafarian movement, and may be seen as a symbol of rebellion against White authority.

The ethnic dimension is a complication of a simple issue. Cannabis is used by some members of all ethnic groups, and strongly condemned by many other members of all ethnic groups. The possession of cannabis is illegal, and its presence cannot be tolerated on wards to which the courts send offenders. It is worth noting that, while the courts regard mental illness as a mitigating factor, and are prepared to recommend treatment rather than punishment, they regard substance misuse as an aggravating factor, deserving of more severe punishment. The principles become clear when considering the analogous case of a drink-driver who has killed or caused serious injury. Any claim to have the right to continue drink-driving would appear grossly irresponsible, even if the person claimed that they had a high tolerance and would not be badly affected by alcohol. The same argument must apply when there is a history of violence due to mental illness, and a patient persists in taking a drug which increases the chances of relapse and further violence.

The ethnic aspects of the problem often obscure this issue in practice. Patients may defend their right to smoke cannabis as part of their culture, demanding a sensitive response on the part of staff. It is not uncommon for staff to debate the question of calling in the police to investigate suspected offences of possession or supply. This response may seem heavy-handed to all patients, but is likely to be particularly resented by members of ethnic minorities. Restrictions on food from outside, in an attempt to prevent the smuggling of cannabis, may be more oppressive for patients whose diet is important to their cultural identity.

These problems are raised, not in the hope of providing any simple answers, but as an illustration of the way in which ethnic differences are a constant theme of work within forensic psychiatry, often complicating questions which are otherwise straightforward. Forensic psychiatry deals with patients who have many grievances against society, some real and others imagined. They often have multiple disadvantages, resulting from their status as both offenders and patients, including social, emotional and economic difficulties. To this list must be added, for many patients, the disadvantages associated with being a member of an ethnic minority. The challenge for forensic psychiatry is to respect the patient's ethnic origin without losing sight of the main task, of treating the mentally disordered offender.

References

COPE, R. & NDEGWA, D. (1990) Ethnic differences in admissions to a regional secure unit. *Journal of Forensic Psychiatry*, **1**, 365–378.

EAST LONDON AND THE CITY HEALTH AUTHORITY (1995) *The Woodley Report*. London: East London and the City Health Authority.

HOME OFFICE (1993) *Prison Statistics: England and Wales 1992*. London: HMSO.

—— & DEPARTMENT OF HEALTH AND SOCIAL SECURITY (1975) *Report of the Committee on Mentally Abnormal Offenders*, Cmnd 6244. London: HMSO.

HOOD, R. (1992) *Race and Sentencing*. Oxford: Clarendon Press.

JONES, G. & BERRY, M. (1986) Regional secure units: the emerging picture. In *Current Issues in Clinical Psychology IV* (ed G. Edwards), pp. 24–42. London: Plenum.

MADEN, A., SWINTON, M. & GUNN, J. (1992) The ethnic origin of women serving a prison sentence. *British Journal of Criminology*, **32**, 218–221.

—— (1993) Crime, culture and ethnicity. *International Review of Psychiatry*, **5**, 281–289.

—— (1995) *Women, Prisons and Psychiatry*. London: Butterworth–Heinemann.

15 Satisfaction with mental health services: issues for ethnic minorities

GRAHAM THORNICROFT, SUE PARKMAN and MIRELIA RUGGERI

Patients' satisfaction with services is both an outcome and a process measure. As early as 1966, Donabedian stated that:

> "...the effectiveness of care in achieving and producing health and satisfaction, as defined for its individual members by a particular society or subculture, is the ultimate validator of the quality of care".

Later, Locker & Dunt (1978) suggested that, particularly in long-term care:

> " ... quality of care can become synonymous with quality of life and satisfaction with care an important component of life satisfaction".

Patients' satisfaction with services can therefore be considered as both dependent and independent variables. As a dependent variable, satisfaction has been thought to be influenced by factors such as subjects' expectations with services, attitudes to life, self-esteem, illness behaviour and previous experience of services. As an independent variable, satisfaction can influence the efficacy of interventions, treatment compliance and service utilisation.

Despite these considerations, service users' views have only recently been seen as a subject relevant to service evaluation. Difficulties in both conceptualisation and assessment have negatively influenced research in this field. Scepticism about psychiatric patients' capability to give rational and meaningful judgments about a service, which are not dominated by their expectations or psychiatric illness, has caused concern about the use of patient satisfaction as a means for evaluating interventions.

This biased view, and the fact that patients' statements are often considered useful only as a basis for making and confirming a diagnosis, have certainly played a major role (Brandon, 1981). A more balanced attitude towards this issue is needed, which combines careful analyses of factors which may interfere with patients' judgments with methodologically sound approaches in order to assess satisfaction with services.

This kind of information about satisfaction may illuminate the results obtained about satisfaction using other variables (such as psychopathology, social functioning, quality of life or burden of relatives); nevertheless, satisfaction cannot substitute for information provided by research using such variables or for professional judgement; rather it is complementary. Indeed, a service user's satisfaction may not necessarily be the only goal of a service, and mental health professionals should not feel threatened by assessing service users' satisfaction or feel obliged to fulfil all patients' requests.

The relevant work in this field has been comprehensively reviewed elsewhere (Atkisson & Pascoe, 1983; Kalman, 1983; Lebow, 1983*a,b*; Lehman & Zastowny, 1983; Pascoe, 1983; Zastowny & Lehman, 1988; Corrigan, 1990; Ricketts, 1992; Ruggeri, 1994). Currently, patient satisfaction is seen as an integral part of health service evaluation (Ruggeri, 1994) and is recommended in Britain by *The Patients' Charter 1991* (Department of Health, 1991) for inclusion in any service evaluation. Satisfaction with health services is also related to future use of those services. If treatment is acceptable to patients, they are more likely to make use of services (Ware *et al*, 1978) and treatment is more likely to be successful (Kalman, 1983). Conversely, dissatisfaction with services may be the reason behind patients discontinuing psychiatric care (Hanson & Rapp, 1992).

Ethnicity and mental health service use

Despite the increasing amount of research looking at ethnic issues, a major difficulty is the lack of validity and consistency both in the terms used and in the definitions of those terms, so hindering the comparison of research findings and the formulation of appropriate questions (McKenzie & Crowcroft, 1994; Hutchinson & McKenzie, 1995). Bhui & Christie (1996) use the term 'Black' to denote all racial and cultural groups whose use of the health services may be affected by the difficulties of social disadvantage and racism. This term will also be used in this chapter. As discussed in Chapters 5 and 6, McGovern & Cope (1991) report that Black patients make different use of psychiatric services compared with White patients. Differences were very small but on every measure Black Caribbean people were less likely to make voluntary contact with health services. This included fewer contacts with general practitioners (GPs) before and at admission, fewer voluntary admissions, more absconding from in-patient wards, more discharges against medical advice and less-regular attendances at out-patient services.

These service satisfaction findings suggest that Black Caribbean patients may find psychiatric services less satisfactory or less relevant to their needs. Broadly speaking, there are three reasons for this: (a) the over-representation of Black Caribbean people in psychiatric hospitals (see Chapter 5 also); (b) concepts of illness which are different to those underpinning the Western psychiatric model (see Chapter 7) and which therefore lead to (c) producing a service which may be inappropriate to the needs of many Black people (see Chapter 22).

Over-representation of Black Caribbean patients in psychiatric hospitals

Higher prevalence rates of schizophrenia have been reported among Black Caribbean immigrants than among the White population (Cochrane & Bal, 1977; Carpenter & Brockington, 1980; Dean *et al*, 1981; Littlewood & Lipsedge, 1981; McGovern & Cope, 1987, 1991; King *et al*, 1994) especially among younger males in whom the rate has been estimated to be up to 14 times higher (Harrison *et al*, 1988; see Tables 1 and 2). In addition, high rates of hospital admission under the Mental Health Act have

TABLE 1
Ethnic differences in reported rates of schizophrenia in USA clinical samples (adapted from Adebimpe, 1994)

Clinical setting	% of admissions		Black : White ratio
	White	Black	
State hospitals	31.5	56.3	1.8
Private hospitals	19.2	35.7	1.8
Non-federal hospitals	22.7	38.0	1.7
Veterans affairs medical centres	26.4	44.5	1.7

TABLE 2
Ethnic differences in reported rates of schizophrenia in UK clinical samples (adapted from Adebimpe, 1994)

Study	Incidence per 10 000 population		Black : White ratio
	Whites	Blacks	
Dean *et al* (1981)			
Male	1.1	3.9	5.0
Female	1.2	3.3	5.3
Cochrane & Bal (1977)[1]			
Male	1.2	5.5	3.3
Female	1.0	5.3	2.8
McGovern & Cope (1987)			
16–29 years	1.4	11.7	8.4
30–60 years	1.1	4.7	4.3
Harrison *et al* (1988)			
16–29 years	2.0	29.1	14.6
30–55 years	1.6	19.7	12.3

1. Further details available from the author upon request.

been reported for Black Caribbean patients, again particularly young males (Rwegellera, 1980; Ineichen *et al*, 1984; Littlewood, 1986; McGovern & Cope, 1987; Harrison *et al*, 1989; Owens *et al*, 1991; Davies *et al*, 1996). Police-referred psychiatric admissions from the Black Caribbean community exceed those from the White community (McGovern & Cope, 1987; Dunn & Fahy, 1990; Pipe *et al*, 1991; Turner *et al*, 1992) as do forensic hospital orders (McGovern & Cope, 1991). Previous research has also found that, independent of diagnosis, Black Caribbean patients are more likely to have contact with the police and forensic services (McGovern & Cope, 1991; also see Chapter 14), are more likely to be treated in intensive care facilities if detained under the Mental Health Act (Moodley & Thornicroft, 1988) and more likely to have been detained in secure units and special hospitals (Francis *et al*, 1989).

Admission rates appear to vary by gender as well as by ethnic group. First admission figures for schizophrenia in Black Caribbean women are 13 times higher than the rate for White women, and are nearly double the rate for Black Caribbean men (McGovern & Cope, 1987). The reasons for this are unclear, but it may be that Black Caribbean women are more often judged by health and social welfare agencies on their capabilities to act as parents. Denial of mental illness in patients admitted to acute psychiatric wards has been found more frequently in African–Caribbean patients (Perkins & Moodley, 1993).

Concepts of illness and mental health services

In Western culture, medicine, religion and psychology are clearly demarcated, whereas in other cultures this is less often the case and a more holistic view of health exists. The Western approach is also somewhat individualist in orientation, placing a special value on individuals having the ability to exercise control in their lives, unlike in some Black communities where the understanding of the self is in relation to the family and community (Rack, 1982). Most views of mental health are likely to incorporate a person's sense of fulfilment and identity, not just as an individual, but also as a part of a group or society. The individual therefore needs to be understood in the relevant political and social context (Fernando, 1991). There is a need to understand this and to plan services which can include family therapy and family involvement (Bhui & Christie, 1996). Fernando (1988) also speaks of the mistake of "colour-blind, culture-blind psychiatry" in which symptoms are viewed objectively, but which takes the individual out of his or her social and cultural context. One study among second-generation African–Caribbean people found that most patients thought that Black day centres would be beneficial (McGovern & Hemmings, 1994).

Aspects of gender

Acceptable degrees of privacy may also vary between cultures. Women's traditional role in some cultures as the primary carer of children has a significant influence on the manner in which distress is manifested and must therefore be taken account of in any treatment package offered. Popular methods of child care and women's perceived roles in the UK cannot be readily assumed to be assigned to Black women, whose socio-cultural roles are likely to place unique expectations upon them and demand the fulfilment of specific obligations (see Chapter 5). The impact on Black women of the interaction of these roles with existing health services has been subject to little research or attention (Bhui & Christie, 1996).

Cultural biases in mental health services

Black Caribbean patients are more likely to be admitted under Section 136 compared with a White population and are less likely to be admitted routinely through their GP (Turner *et al*, 1992). Thus, the higher rates of compulsory admission to psychiatric facilities and the differential use of treatments between different racial groups continue to be a matter of importance. It therefore appears from this evidence that the health needs of Black people may often be compromised; they are already a disadvantaged group which has faced difficulties of immigration and its consequences and they more often suffer psychiatric disorders (Cochrane & Bal, 1977; London, 1986).

British studies have suggested that Black people are less likely to receive diagnoses of anxiety or depression in primary care (see Chapter 7). This is paradoxical, as causal factors also applicable to anxiety and depressive disorders are among the socio-cultural explanations put forward to account for higher rates of schizophrenia among Black people (Lloyd, 1993); consistent with this hypothesis are studies indicating higher rates of anxiety and depressive disorders among Black primary care attenders (Kiev, 1965; also see Chapter 7). Burke (1984) suggests that non-recognition by GPs is responsible and reported that GPs failed to make a diagnosis in 21% of Black patients and 13% of White patients identified as ill by a screening instrument (Bhui & Christie, 1996).

Implications for research on service satisfaction

Substantial differences have been demonstrated in the pattern of contacts with psychiatric services of patients from different ethnic groups, especially between those who are White and Black Caribbean. These differences spread across most aspects of specialist mental health service provision. So far, these are largely expert-reported differences, or are aggregated data from in-patient service contacts. It is striking that information is largely absent in the psychiatric literature from the perspective of the patients themselves, of whatever ethnic group. Since types of contact with services vary so much, it is reasonable to hypothesise that service users' views of services prior to, during and after such contact may also differ substantially by ethnic group. These views may then affect how such people use services in future. In this way the experiences that patients accumulate from using services progress in ways which reflect their expectations, satisfaction, perception of illness and 'harder' aspects such as the number of admissions, particularly those which are compulsory. The ways in which such psychiatric 'careers' develop in relation to ethnic group, and their implications for how services can be sensitised to ethnic issues, are yet to be properly understood.

References

ADEBIMPE, V. (1994) Race, racism and epidemiological surveys. *Hospital and Community Psychiatry*, **45**, 27–31.

ATKISSON, C. C. & PASCOE, G. C. (eds) (1983) Patient satisfaction in health and mental health services. In *Evaluation & Program Planning*, Vol. 6, special issue, pp. 19–31. New York: Pergamon Press.

BHUI, K. & CHRISTIE, Y. (1996) Purchasing mental health services for Black communities. In *Commissioning Mental Health Services* (eds G. Thornicroft & G. Strathdee), pp 215–230. London: HMSO.

BRANDON, D. (1981) *Voices of Experience; Consumer Perspectives of Psychiatric Treatment*. London: MIND.

BURKE, A. W. (1984) Racism and psychological disturbance among West Indians in Britain. *International Journal of Social Psychiatry*, **30**, 50–68.

CARPENTER, L. & BROCKINGTON, I. F. (1980) A study of mental illness in Asians, West Indians and Africans living in Manchester. *British Journal of Psychiatry*, **137**, 201–205.

COCHRANE, R. & BAL, J. (1977) Mental illness in immigrants to England and Wales: An analysis of mental hospital admissions, 1971. *Social Psychiatry*, **12**, 25–35.

CORRIGAN, P. W. (1990) Consumer satisfaction with institutional and community care. *Community Mental Health Journal*, **26**, 151–165.

DAVIES, S., THORNICROFT, G., LEESE, M., *et al* (1996) Ethnic differences in the risk of compulsory psychiatric admission among representative cases of psychosis in London. *British Medical Journal*, **312**, 533–537.

DEAN, G., WALSH, D., DOWNING, H., *et al* (1981) First admissions of native-born and immigrants to psychiatric hospitals in south-east England 1976. *British Journal of Psychiatry*, **139**, 506–512.

DEPARTMENT OF HEALTH (1991) *The Patients' Charter 1991*. London: Department of Health.

DONABEDIAN, A. (1966) Evaluating the quality of medical care. *Milibank Memorial Fund*, **44**, 166–203.

DUNN, J. & FAHY, T. (1990) Police admissions to a psychiatric hospital. Demographic and clinical differences between ethnic groups. *British Journal of Psychiatry*, **156**, 373–378.

FERNANDO, S. (1988) *Race & Culture in Psychiatry*. London: Tavistock/Routledge.

—— (1991) *Mental Health, Race and Culture*. London: Macmillan.

FRANCIS, E., DAVID, J., JOHNSON, N., *et al* (1989) Black people and psychiatry in the UK. An alternative to institutional care. *Psychiatric Bulletin*, **13**, 482–485.

HANSON, J. G. & RAPP, C. A. (1992) Families' perceptions of community mental health programs for their relatives with a severe mental illness. *Community Mental Health Journal*, **28**, 181–195.

HARRISON, G., OWENS, D., HOLTON, A., *et al* (1988) A prospective study of severe mental disorder in Afro-Caribbean patients. *Psychological Medicine*, **18**, 643–657.

——, HOLTON, A., NEILSON, D., *et al* (1989) Severe mental disorder in Afro-Caribbean patients: some social, demographic and service factors. *Psychological Medicine*, **19**, 683–696.

HUTCHINSON, G. & MCKENZIE, G. (1995) What is the Afro-Caribbean implication for psychiatric research. *Psychiatric Bulletin*, **19**, 700–702.

INEICHEN, B., HARRISON, G. & MORGAN, H. G. (1984) Psychiatric hospital admissions in Bristol. I. Geographical and ethnic factors. *British Journal of Psychiatry*, **145**, 600–661.

KALMAN, T. P. (1983) An overview of patient satisfaction with psychiatric treatment. *Hospital and Community Psychiatry*, **34**, 48–54.

KIEV, A. (1965) Psychiatric morbidity of West Indian immigrants in an urban group practice. *British Journal of Psychiatry*, **111**, 51–56.

KING, M., COKER, E., LEAVEY, G., *et al* (1994) Incidence of psychotic illness in London: comparison of ethnic groups. *British Medical Journal*, **309**, 1115–1119.

LEBOW, J. L. (1983*a*) Client satisfaction with mental health treatment: methodological considerations in assessment. *Evaluation Review*, **7**, 729–752.

—— (1983*b*) Similarities and differences between mental health and health care evaluation studies assessing consumer satisfaction. *Evaluation & Program Planning*, **6**, 237–245.

LEHMAN, A. F. & ZASTOWNY, T. R. (1983) Patient satisfaction with mental health services; a metanalysis to establish norms. *Evaluation & Program Planning*, **6**, 265–274.

LITTLEWOOD, R. (1986) Ethnic minorities and the Mental Health Act. Patterns of explanation. *Psychiatric Bulletin*, **10**, 306–308.

—— & LIPSEDGE, M. (1981) Some social and phenomenological characteristics of psychotic immigrants. *Psychological Medicine*, **11**, 289–302.

LLOYD, K. (1993) Depression and anxiety among Afro-Caribbean general practice attenders in Britain. *International Journal of Social Psychiatry*, **39**, 1–9.

LOCKER, D. & DUNT, D. (1978) Theoretical and methodological issues in sociological studies of consumer satisfaction with medical care. *Social Science & Medicine*, **12**, 283–292.

LONDON, M. (1986) Mental illness among immigrants in the United Kingdom. *British Journal of Psychiatry*, **149**, 265–273.

McGOVERN, D. & COPE, R. (1987) The compulsory detention of males of different ethnic groups, with special reference to offender patients. *British Journal of Psychiatry*, **150**, 505–512.

—— & —— (1991) Second generation of Afro-Caribbeans and young Whites with a first admission diagnosis of schizophrenia. *Social Psychiatry and Psychiatric Epidemiology*, **26**, 95–99.

—— & HEMMINGS, P. (1994) A follow-up of second generation Afro-Caribbeans and White British with a first admission diagnosis of schizophrenia: attitudes to mental illness and psychiatric services of patients and relatives. *Social Science & Medicine*, **38**, 117–127.

McKENZIE, K. & CROWCROFT, N. (1994) Race, ethnicity, culture and science. *British Medical Journal*, **309**, 285–287.

MOODLEY, P. & THORNICROFT, G. (1988) Ethnic group and compulsory detention. *Medicine, Science and the Law*, **28**, 324–328.

OWENS, D., HARRISON, G. & BOOT, D. (1991) Ethnic factors in voluntary and compulsory admissions. *Psychological Medicine*, **21**, 185–196.

PASCOE, G. C. (1983) Patient satisfaction in primary health care: a literature review and analysis. *Evaluation & Program Planning*, **6**, 185–210.

PERKINS, R. F. & MOODLEY, P. (1993) Perception of problems in psychiatric inpatients: denial, race and service usage. *Social Psychiatry and Psychiatric Epidemiology*, **28**, 189–193.

PIPE, R., BATH, A., MATTHEWS, B., *et al* (1991) Section 136 and African/Afro-Caribbean minorities. *International Journal of Social Psychiatry*, **37**, 14–23.

RACK, P. (1982) *Race, Culture and Mental Disorder*. London: Tavistock.

RICKETTS, T. (1992) Consumer satisfaction surveys in mental health. *British Journal of Nursing*, **1**, 523–527.

RUGGERI, M. (1994) Patients' and relatives' satisfaction with psychiatric services: the state of the art of its measurement. *Social Psychiatry and Psychiatric Epidemiology*, **29**, 212–227.

RWEGELLERA, G. G. C. (1980) Differential use of psychiatric services by West Indians, West Africans and English in London. *British Journal of Psychiatry*, **137**, 428–432.

TURNER, T. H., NESS, M. N. & IMISON, C. T. (1992) Mentally disordered persons found in public places. Diagnostic and social aspects of police referrals (Section 136). *Psychological Medicine*, **22**, 765–774.

WARE, J. E., DAVIES-AVERY, A. & STEWART, A. I. (1978) The measurement and meaning of patient satisfaction. *Health and Medical Care Services Review*, **1**, 2–15.

ZASTOWNY, T. R. & LEHMAN, A. F. (1988) Patient satisfaction with mental health services. *Quality Revision Bulletin*, **14**, 284–289.

16 Joint working between the public and purchasing authorities to determine mental health information needs

CAROL M. GRANT-PEARCE and JULIA DEANE

Purchasing authorities, that is, health authorities and Family Health Service Authorities, are seen to have a major role in determining health needs so as to ensure that health services available to the public are equitable, comprehensive, efficient, effective and accessible. However, only after the public has gained access to services can we discuss whether services are appropriate or sensitive to their needs and expectations. One of the many factors which can influence accessibility to services is information. Minority group involvement is required in order to determine what information they need to support their mental health needs.

Background

The dictionary definition (Hanks, 1989) of accessibility includes: "easy to approach, enter or use, available, understandable". At central level within the Department of Health, the importance of information in accessing services has been acknowledged by the *Patients' Charter And You* (Department of Health, 1995), which states that every individual has the right to receive detailed information on local health services, and includes information on the standards of service that can be expected. The NHS Executive Mental Health Task Force (1994) highlighted as a priority for purchasers and providers the need for:

"Improvements in consultation, communication and access information ... to bring back communities including users and carers into the planning structure".

The communities mentioned represent diverse constituencies served by the NHS. Barnes & Wistow (1994) divide the community into three groups, according to the way they use mental health services: (a) those who use services directly – whether voluntary or involuntary, short- or long-term, as individuals or as groups; (b) those who are involved in mental health services indirectly, for example, carers; and (c) those who are potential users, such as citizens. This categorisation of the public allows us to see more clearly the potential mental health information needs of the public. Information is required for those who use services directly, indirectly and potential users. Barnes & Wistow (1994) challenge professional dominance over deciding the needs of users, by advocating that purchasers should give users a more meaningful involvement in the process.

Klein (1984) reviewed public participation in health issues by problematising it as a debate between paternalism of health professionals in deciding public needs versus active public involvement in deciding what their needs are. He highlights the conflict between the broader social model of needs assessment used by the public to support health gain, with the medical model usually used by medical professionals in purchasing units. The former acknowledges that services other than health services are needed to address mental health needs. The latter tend to confine their policy responses to health services.

Klein and Barnes & Wistow are part of the school of thought which sees public participation in deciding information needs as beneficial to improving access and sensitivity of services. They acknowledge the right of users to have an input in decisions that ultimately affect them. The oppostion, which still predominates in many purchasing authorities, believe that 'health experts' know what is best for service users, and do not recognise the invaluable knowledge contained within user groups.

The National Health Service (NHS) Community Care Act 1990 and the document *Local Voices* (NHS Management Executive, 1992) have provided some impetus within purchasing organisations to involve the public in identifying health needs. By listening to what users have to say and involving them in health issues, services can be made more accessible and appropriate. Although a step in the right direction, this is an approach from the top working downwards, instigated by the NHS Executive.

Refugees are a section of the public who have clear information needs about NHS mental health services and also other, non-health services. A study was instigated by the Brixton Refugee Health Project which addressed the mental health information needs of refugee groups (see also Chapter 2).

Brixton Refugee Health Project

Background

The Brixton Challenge wards contain 58 000 people, approximately a quarter of Lambeth's population. More than a quarter of the residents were born outside the UK. Many of these people do not access mental health services when there is a clinical need. There may be a range of reasons for this, but one is the quality and paucity of information about such services. In this chapter the term refugee is used to embrace refugees, asylum seekers and those with "exceptional leave to remain" for humanitarian reasons (this given at the discretion of the Home Office).

A survey performed between July and December 1994 used a structured questionnaire and discussion groups to obtain information about the needs of refugees in primary care. Refugee volunteers were recruited to interview a convenience sample (the nearest and most convenient people to act as respondents; Robson, 1995) of the refugee population from 12 language-speaking groups in the Brixton Challenge area of Lambeth.

Results

Profile of respondents

Of the 270 survey respondents aged between 18 and 75 years, 53% were male, 45% were female and 2% did not give their gender. The mother tongue of respondents was wide ranging (Fig. 1). Seventy refugees took part in the discussion groups: 54% discussed information needs and the rest mental health service needs.

Mental illness

Forty-five per cent of respondents in the survey felt that they had developed mental health problems since arrival in the UK and 10% felt that they already had mental health problems before arrival. Reasons suggested by discussion groups for this increase in morbidity included: uncertainty about their immigration status, concern about relatives in their home country and housing and employment

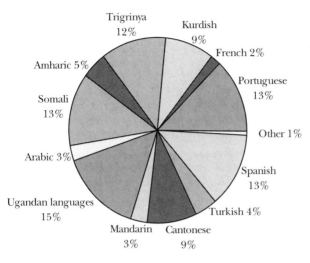

FIG. 1
Languages spoken by respondents

uncertainties. Older respondents were more likely to say they were depressed than their younger counterparts.

Sources of mental health support and information

The type of mental health support sought by refugees included formal and informal support from statutory and voluntary agencies (Fig. 2). Respondents tended to use general practioners (GPs), who they felt were sympathetic to their needs and were more likely to give information on the range of mental health support services available. These GPs usually had refugee hostels in their area or had staff who spoke appropriate languages. However, respondents also felt that many GPs were unaware of refugee community support groups in their area who could provide social support. Friends, relatives and community groups were other significant sources of support and the main source of information about the health services (Fig. 3). What is of interest and of concern is the proportion of respondents who sought no help when they had mental health problems.

The type of information that respondents wanted about mental health services included:

(a) how the mental health system is organised;
(b) what services are available;
(c) where services are located;

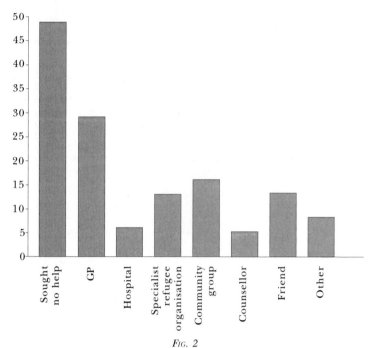

Fig. 2
Where help was sought for mental health support (base=139)

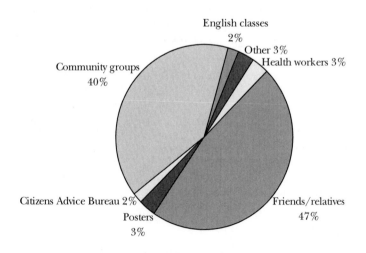

Fig. 3
How people were informed about health services

(d) what alternative types of treatment are available;
(e) what to expect at consultation;
(f) patients' rights under the Mental Health Act.

Other issues were seen as having higher priority than health issues soon after arrival in the UK. They were centred around housing, immigration, employment, education and welfare support. Easy access to information about these services was thought to be important in alleviating much anxiety and stress. Although just under half (48%) of the respondents claimed that their English comprehension enabled them to understand most of what was written and spoken, interpreting services were felt to be needed by 52% of respondents. In 75% of cases relatives, friends and community groups acted as interpreters in health situations.

As an indicator of the respondents' knowledge about health services, they were asked what number they would ring for an emergency ambulance. Twenty-three per cent of respondents did not know the correct number.

How to address information needs

Those who took part in discussion groups made suggestions on how their information needs regarding mental health services could be addressed. These are:

(a) Employing and training people from refugee community groups to communicate information about health and other services available and their rights to use them.
(b) Development of health education literature in the main refugee languages.
(c) Strengthening links between statutory mental health services and the specialist organisations working with refugees.
(d) Using a wider range of community venues to disseminate information, for example social clubs, refugee training and enterprise centres, religious venues, creches and large gatherings such as national celebration days.
(e) Interpreting via health advocates/health interpreters.
(f) Health venues also providing information about other services, for example, education and housing.

Conclusions

Despite the limitations of this study, such as the small sample size and issues concerning the representativeness of the sample, certain interesting points were raised.

More community venues need to be utilised to aid the dissemination and transmission of information about health services and support. Refugee community groups appear to be an invaluable resource, and health advocates from those communities who speak the appropriate languages have a useful role to play.

It is of concern that there were a number of people who did not seek help for mental health problems. This begs the question of whether or not this also is a feature within the general population. A study by Gillam *et al* (1989), on consultation rates in general practice for mental disorders, noted reduced consultation rates for anxiety and depression in all immigrant groups.

General practice is usually the first point of contact with the NHS for most refugees; it serves as a useful venue for information and advice (both written and verbal) to be provided about mental health and welfare support services in a locality.

Purchasing authorities and other statutory agencies have a role to play in ensuring that adequate and appropriate information is easily available about mental health services, and other services that could be used to address the mental health needs of refugees. Written or verbal information, whatever the language, should be uncomplicated. It is not sufficient to translate directly from an English version (Smith, 1992); emphasis should be placed on refugee community involvement in producing information so that it is appropriate to their needs.

This study looked at ways to improve access to primary care services for refugees in the Brixton area and found a clear need for the information needs of refugees to be addressed. Public participation in developing information is needed to ensure that the information produced is meaningful and appropriate to assist refugees accessing mental health and other services.

Acknowledgements

We thank Brixton Challenge (the main funder of the Brixton Refugee Health Project), Lambeth, Southwark and Lewisham Health Commission and all those who took part in this project.

References

Barnes, M. & Wistow, G. (1994) Achieving a strategy for user involvement in community care. *Health and Social Care*, **2**, 347–356.

Department of Health (1995) *Patients' Charter and You*. Leeds: Department of Health.

Gillam, S. J., Jarman, B., White, P., *et al* (1989) Ethnic differences in consultation rates in urban general practice. *British Medical Journal*, **299**, 953–957.

HANKS, P. (ed.)(1989) *Collins Concise Dictionary Plus,* 1st edn. London: William Collins & Co.

KLEIN, R. (1984) The politics of participation. In *Public Participation in Health: Towards a Clearer View* (eds R. Maxwell & N. Weaver). London: King's Fund Publishing Office.

NHS EXECUTIVE (1992) *Local Voices: the Views of Local People in Purchasing for Health.* Leeds: NHS Executive.

NHS EXECUTIVE MENTAL HEALTH TASK FORCE (1994) *Black Mental Health – A Dialogue for Change.* Leeds: NHSE.

SMITH, T. (1992) Information for patients. *British Medical Journal,* **305,** 1242.

ROBSON, C. (1995) *Real World Research: A Resource for Social Scientists and Practitioner–Researchers.* Oxford: Blackwell.

17 Culture, ethnicity and mental health. A purchaser's perspective on the mental health of Black and other ethnic minority groups

PETER GLUCKMAN

Lambeth, Southwark and Lewisham Health Commission in south London provide services for nearly 750 000 people. The geographical area has a significant proportion of Black and minority ethnic groups living there. There has been recognition for some time of the difficulties faced by Black and other minority ethnic communities in relation to mental health. If mental disorder can be said to be determined by society, then cultural issues will clearly impact upon our understanding of what constitutes being mentally disordered, and the prevailing culture will be used to judge this state. Goldberg has commented on this subject (Chapter 3), but the issues are complex and do not allow for quick and easy solutions.

The complexity affects all NHS purchasers. Their role, in consultation with service providers and other partners, is to assess the (mental health) needs of their population, to define and to put in place the services required to meet that need and then to evaluate and monitor quality of care within an agreed cost. This process evolves continually as population need, clinical knowledge and financial frameworks change over time.

This chapter relates to the health authority covering the three southeast, socially deprived inner London boroughs of Lambeth, Southwark and Lewisham. The official census population is 730 000 of which 26% are from a very diverse range of Black and minority ethnic communities. The actual population is estimated at 860 000. The difference between official and local estimates of residents is explained by those who decided not to register with the census and the excluded populations, for example, refugees, asylum seekers, homeless people and young adults living temporarily in the area.

National Health Service reforms in 1991 and 1997

The purchaser/provider split in the structure of the National Health Service (NHS) introduced by the Conservative government in 1991 and maintained by the new Labour government in 1997 might be expected to assist in meeting the mental health needs of Black and minority ethnic groups. It allows commissioners to gather information from literature and needs assessment studies to inform purchasing of services that are appropriate to these communities. However, commissioners vary in their capability and willingness to take on such work. For those who work in the inner cities, it is clearly a vital area and one that cannot simply be ignored. The *Income and Wealth Report* (Joseph Rowntree Foundation Enquiry Group, 1995) focused attention on the widening gap between the rich and poor, as in the inner cities extreme deprivation and affluence sit alongside each other. In some areas nearly two-thirds of young Black men do not have employment. To some extent there appears to be a correlation between economic deprivation and levels of morbidity in mental health. It does not seem to be a coincidence that young Black men constitute a large proportion of the patients in local services; and Leff (see Chapter 5) has illustrated material links between unemployment and mental well-being.

A joint initiative by the King's Fund Centre, the Mental Health Task Force and the Prince of Wales' Advisory Group (Wilson *et al*, 1993) on *Mental Health and Britain's Black Communities* has been published. This was followed by the Task Force programme of consultation with Black mental health groups and organisations. *Black Mental Health – A Dialogue for Change* (NHS Executive Mental Health Task Force, 1994) was then published. It sets out the following key areas for purchasers to address:

(a) development of the role of the Black non-statutory sector;
(b) improvement of consultations, communication and the accessibility of information;
(c) development of closer relationships with community forums;
(d) acknowledgement of the work and experience of Black professionals in statutory organisations.

It is important to ascertain how these priorities correlate with those identified locally during the work undertaken to inform the Health Commission's five-year mental health strategy *With Need in Mind* (Lambeth, Southwark & Lewisham Health Commission, 1994).

Audit

A full audit of NHS services by independent Black organisations will be undertaken, although some limited work in this area has already taken place and services have been adjusted in response.

Meetings

It is intended that general practitioners (GPs) and Black groups should meet on both a Black community and authority-wide basis, although there have been a number of initiatives by individual practices, for example, the Wells Park Health Project. Their report (Wells Park Health Project, 1994) sets out a number of recommendations including: having a Black counsellor based at the practice; work around family therapy; helping people who commit self-harm with their identity problems and providing therapeutic help.

Specialist support services run by Black providers

Three local Black non-statutory organisations have been supported: the African–Caribbean Mental Health Association (in Lambeth, Southwark and Lewisham), Isis in Lewisham and Brixton Circle (Fanon) in Lambeth. All of these provide specific, culturally appropriate services to their communities. However, voluntary-sector projects can sometimes run into trouble with tension between management committees and paid workers, and these difficulties have been experienced at a local level (see Chapter 20). In addition, there has been investment by the health authority, by local boroughs and by organisations such as London Borough's Grants Unit in Asian projects (principally aimed at people from the Indian subcontinent), Vietnamese projects and refugee projects. There is a need, however, to create financial stability for these groups. Too often, their money has been derived from 'soft' sources and has to be renewed each year, in a number of streams and from a number of purchasers. Parity must be created for Black groups offering services.

We should also remember that the informal support systems which operate, sometimes in spite of the statutory sector rather than with its support, are vitally important.

Therapy services

Much of the work undertaken by specialist Black providers is in providing therapeutic interventions and strategies which, for reasons

Box 1
Service usage: over-representation

Black people are over-represented in:
- Secure units.
- Special hospitals.
- Intensive care units.
- Use of physical treatments.
- Use of electroconvulsive therapy and depot drug treatment.
- 'Challenging behaviour' units.
- Admissions involving a police presence.
- Admissions by section of the Mental Health Act.

that are not entirely clear, are not always offered by mainstream NHS organisations to Black patients as often as they are to White patients.

Anti-racist training

It is important that Black people are not forced to use only specialised 'Black services'. It is appropriate for some people, on occasion, to be in the care of those services, but this does not mean that they will never need to make use of generic statutory services.

The establishment of specialist services for Black people and people from other ethnic minorities does not let the statutory sector off the hook. NHS providers must find ways to improve access to services for these groups and to attempt to ensure that the services they offer are non-threatening and culturally appropriate (see Chapters 15, 19 and 23).

It is important to discover the scale of the problem and how the issues present themselves in service usage terms. Leff (Chapter 5) has demonstrated the importance of epidemiology and using acquired knowledge and understanding to commission services.

Black people are massively over-represented in secure services; some 70–80% of Lambeth, Southwark and Lewisham's local medium secure population is made up of young Black men (see Chapter 14). This is true for special hospitals, intensive care units and 'challenging behaviour' units. Black people are more likely to be sectioned. In a local study, *Psychiatric Research in Service Measurement* (PRiSM, 1994), 81% of Black Caribbean service users born in the UK had been 'sectioned' during their illness (compulsorily placed under section of the Mental Health Act 1983), compared with 54% of White people in the survey. Black people are more likely to be delivered to hospital by the police. They are more likely to be given physical treatments, including electroconvulsive therapy (ECT), and are more likely to be given depot drug therapy. Box 1 summarises this over-representation phenomenon.

The corollary of this over-representation at the most acute end of services is under-representation of Black people in other parts of the service (see Chapter 15).

Day care services are less likely to be accessed by Black people, psychological therapies are less likely to be offered to them, and there is a lack of access to services at the primary care level. Some Black people report high levels of dissatisfaction with GP services, including racist attitudes and feelings that they are unwelcome. It has been argued that this creates a vicious circle. Lack of access to early intervention and primary services leads to a worsening of condition to the point at which hospital admission is required. However, because of their experiences of hospital services, Black people are not willing to be admitted and so they are sectioned, picked up by the police and delivered or, in the more extreme cases, arrested for some offence and passed on to forensic services.

Box 2
Innovative responses locally in Lambeth, Southwark & Lewisham

Black alternatives to hospital project – Ipamo (Lambeth)
● Initially funded by LIG.
● Planned by the local NHS provider.
● Planned in collaboration with local Black agencies
● Service provision to be by a non-statutory Black agency/agencies.
● Wide range of services available, including crisis intervention and day care, all of which are community-based.

Black Mental Health Centre (Lewisham)
● A joint approach by the Health Commission, Lewisham & Guy's Mental Health NHS Trust, the Borough and a local Black agency (Isis).
● The centre has its own premises.
● Stabilisation of 'soft' funding.

Forensic audit
● By a Black group – the Afro-Caribbean Mental Health Association.
● A report was prepared.
● Sectorisation of adult mental health services.
● Development of contracts with local voluntary organisations.
● Longer-term contracts for NHS mental health trusts and voluntary organisations.
● 'Pump priming' (providing start-up funding for community-based services before they are supported by mainstream funding) and evaluating extended mental health services in primary care settings.

Improvements

The NHS Executive Mental Health Task Force (1994) reported on a number of innovative services. Box 2 shows three of the local innovations. A Lambeth project called Ipamo was funded by the London Implementation Group (LIG) following the Secretary of State's announcement, in April 1994, of additional funding for mental health schemes. This followed the publication of the report into the care and treatment of Christopher Clunis (Ritchie *et al*, 1994). It was intended that the Ipamo project would move to mainstream funding after the three-year LIG support period. The project was planned by a partnership committee which included the health authority, two local mental health trusts (Lambeth Healthcare NHS Trust and the Bethlem & Maudsley NHS Trust), the King's Fund, Lambeth Social Services and a number of local Black agencies and community organisations.

There are two main strands to the services provided by Ipamo (see Box 3): a crisis and assessment centre, with 10 beds, living areas and therapy rooms; and a family and community outreach service which provides, in addition to daytime facilities, a three-bed family suite and respite beds for carers. The intention was for Ipamo to be managed and operated by a consortium of Black organisations.

In all of these local initiatives, Lambeth, Southwark & Lewisham Health Authority has attempted to use mainstream funding and to make these services an integral part of local service provision. It is vital that this process is completed and that Black organisations have the same levels of stability as NHS providers.

Box 3
Alternative to hospital for the African and Caribbean communities – Ipamo

Facilities at Ipamo House (a crisis and assessment centre)
- Five beds (male) with bathroom, toilets, shower room.
- Five beds (female) with bathroom, toilets, shower room.
- Kitchen/living room, quiet room, sleeping-in room, dining room, two therapy rooms, an assessment suite and a staff toilet and shower.

A family and community outreach service, including day facilities and respite for carers, containing
- Family suite – a three-bed self-contained unit.
- Four beds to provide respite for carers.
- Kitchen/diner, lounge, bathroom, toilet, staff office, reception area, two consultation rooms, a crèche, management office, training room and staff toilet.

Box 4
Areas for further work

With the Vietnamese community:
- Currently there is only limited investment in local groups.
- Mainly joint finance/soft funding.
- A local study (Deptford, Lewisham) has shown that this community has many needs in the health care area.

With the Asian community:
- Continuing support of two local projects.
- Lack of access to services has been acknowledged as a major issue.
- Women are a priority group (there is a higher ratio of suicides among young Asian women).

With the Latin American community:
- Very little is known about this community; there is a need for research.
- The size of the community is growing, therefore identification of their needs is important.

With refugees:
- Many are from the Horn of Africa, central Africa and former Yugoslavia – high levels of stress and trauma from effects of war torture are common.
- Some refugees are suspicious of government agencies.

Efforts have been concentrated locally on the Black African and Caribbean communities as they are the major service users and represent the largest ethnic minority groups in south London. However, there is a clear need to meet the expectations of other, smaller communities (see Box 4). The Vietnamese community has recently become established in the UK, and local studies have identified major needs which have not been met. People from the Indian subcontinent, especially women, are often unable to access services or discuss cultural issues concerned with the acceptance of mental illness. The size of the Latin American and eastern European communities is also increasing in the UK, and their members do not use available services. In the USA, attempts have been made to reach this community using comics written in both Spanish and English to try to educate this community about health care, albeit with limited success (see Chapter 19).

In 1996, a major shift in commissioning and purchasing of health care services occurred. Under the Health Authorities Act 1995 all district health and family health service authorities were abolished and new combined health authorities were established. They cover primary, community, mental health, secondary and specialist hospital services. The parallel extension of GP fund-holding was an element of the government's broader strategy to move towards a primary care-led NHS (NHS Executive, 1994*a*), to secure an increased emphasis on improving clinical effectiveness and to base decision-making on sound evidence (NHS Executive, 1994*b*).

Primary care and general practice will increasingly be in the forefront of deciding what mental health services should exist. The new government announced the end of GP fund-holding in its present form in its White paper *The New NHS* (Department of Health, 1997). It views the primary health care team as the building block of the NHS, with the GP at its centre (see Chapter 19). Primary care groups (which will come into being in April 1999) will include all general practices along with community nurses, health authority representatives, social services and lay people.

The potential impact of the continuing changes to the NHS on mental health services for Black people is still not fully known. My concern is that just as the system (with all its strengths and weaknesses) begins to settle down, and as the needs of Black and ethnic minority groups become prominent on the agenda, restructuring will divert attention away from them. Goldberg (Chapter 3) has stressed the importance of understanding and improving the relationship between primary health care teams and the ethnic minorities. In 1988 the Minister of Health launched the National Association of Health Authorities (1988) excellent report *Action Not Words*, which described a strategy to improve health services for ethnic minority groups. It was quickly lost in the restructuring prompted by *Working for Patients* (Department of Health, 1989).

The new emphasis on partnership-making in the new Labour governments's policy documents, *The New NHS* (Department of Health, 1997) and *Our Healthier Nation* (Department of Health, 1998*b*) means that the language of the internal market will not divert the NHS towards introspective posturing. We must remember what the system is trying to achieve. This aim has a better chance of success with the development of *Health Improvement Programmme* (Department of Health, 1998*a*), which require all health and social care services to assess jointly the needs of Black and minority communities (among others). For Black and other ethnic minority communities, good access to primary care, effective relationships between GPs, psychiatrists and the rest of the mental health professions, and much better collaboration between the NHS, local authorities and the voluntary sector should bring commissioners and providers together.

To understand the complexity and sensitivies of how culture and ethnicity relate to mental health, and to respond in the right way, purchasers have to develop sufficient expertise and understanding of the factors involved. We must be able to complement, and be able to interact effectively with, specialist providers. Purchasers can bring an important and different perspective to the topic; they have an overview of this complex system as a whole, while providers do not always see the whole picture. The purchasing element of service provision is just one uniquely positioned part of the process.

Much work still needs to be done. Needs assessment must be carried out at general practice primary care group level as well as at a wider population level. New and innovative services must be commissioned for the ethnic minority population. A long and complex agenda now stretches before us if we are to utilise the benefits that the new system creates: by retaining the purchaser–provider relationship in the context of partnership working and by term service agreements (contacts). We must endeavour to bring about real changes and effective service provision for the ethnic minorities in the area of mental health, whatever structures are given to us to work within and however they change.

References

DEPARTMENT OF HEALTH (1989) *Working for Patients. The Health Service – Caring for the 1990s.* London: HMSO.
—— (1997) *The New NHS: Modern Dependable,* Cm 3807. London: HMSO.
—— (1998a) *Health Improvement Programme: Planning for Better Health and Better Health Care,* HSC 1998/167: LAC(98) 23. London: Department of Health.
—— (1998b) *Our Healthier Nation: A Contract for Health,* Cm 3852. London: HMSO.
JOSEPH ROWNTREE FOUNDATION ENQUIRY GROUP (1995) *Inquiry into Income and Wealth,* Vol. 1. London: Joseph Rowntree Foundation.
LAMBETH, SOUTHWARK & LEWISHAM HEALTH COMMISSION (1994) *With Need in Mind – A Five-Year Commissioning Strategy for Mental Health Services in South-East London, 1994/95 to 1998/99.* London: Lambeth, Southwark & Lewisham Health Commission.
NATIONAL ASSOCIATION OF HEALTH AUTHORITIES (1988) *Action Not Words – A Strategy to Improve Health Services for Black Minority Ethnic Groups.* Birmingham: National Association of Health Authorities.
NHS EXECUTIVE (1994a) *Developing NHS Purchasing and GP Fund-Holding. Towards a Primary Care Led NHS,* EL(94)79. Leeds: NHS Executive.
—— (1994b) *Improving the Effectiveness of the NHS,* EL(94)74. London: NHS Executive.
NHS EXECUTIVE MENTAL HEALTH TASK FORCE (1994) *Black Mental Health – A Dialogue for Change.* Leeds: NHS Executive.
PRiSM (1994) *Psychiatric Research in Service Measurement.* London: PRiSM.
RITCHIE, J., DICK, D. & LINGHAM, R. (1994) *Report of the Inquiry into the Care and Treatment of Christopher Clunis.* London: North East Thames and South East Thames Regional Health Authorities & HMSO.
WELLS PARK HEALTH PROJECT (1994) *Report of the African–Caribbean Development Health Worker,* (ed. T. Sinclair). London: Wells Park Health Project.
WILSON, M., NHS MANAGEMENT EXECUTIVE, MENTAL HEALTH TASK FORCE, et al (1993) *Mental Health and Britain's Black Communities.* London: King's Fund Centre.

18 The National Health Service and ethnicity: services for Black patients

JANET LA GRENADE

This chapter is concerned mainly with people of African–Caribbean and African descent. This is a very heterogeneous grouping and to include other ethnic groups, such as those from the Indian subcontinent, would do great injustice to these populations. The following observations are a result of my year-long sabbatical in inner-city London.

African–Caribbean people have been present in Britain since the era of the slave trade. Significant numbers of West Indians fought in the First and Second World Wars. In the 1950s and 1960s there was a large influx of migrants from the Caribbean to the UK. Many were actively recruited to fill underserved areas of the economy and the civil service, whereas others came expecting to find jobs and working conditions to improve the quality of their lives. In the main, their perspective was that they were coming to the 'mother country' – a place with perhaps an inhospitable climate, but a place which, because of their education and socialisation as members of the British Empire, they expected to feel at home in. Family units were severely disturbed in this process as many individuals came alone and passages were paid by the joint endeavours of many family members. The expectation was that as soon as it was economically feasible other family members would join them in the UK.

It was also expected that, while migrants would do any job to keep bread on the table, the purpose of the migration was to create a higher standard of living for their children. In Caribbean societies this generally is achieved via the educational system, where increased access to education meant that, for those who excelled, social mobility was almost guaranteed.

The difficulties of migrant children in the school system have been documented (Barker, 1973; Cochrane, 1979; also see Chapters 9 and 10). A disproportionate number of Black children found themselves labelled 'educationally subnormal' and were given education and career guidance appropriate to this ascription. Many came of age in a time of economic decline, massive unemployment and rising nationalism. Black discontent erupted in the summer riots of 1981 in Brixton, London, which were later echoed in other urban centres throughout the UK. Four factors were intially felt to be important in causing the riots: economic gloom, an urban setting, a community and a provoking incident were felt to have triggered the riots. Reasearch by an ethnic study group (Bhat *et al*, 1984) concluded that disadvantage and race were factors of equal importance.

Black perceptions of mental health services

Within the Black community, there is an almost palpable feeling of anger towards mental health services, psychiatrists and other service providers. This becomes obvious in formal conference settings or informal gatherings when the subject is raised. For example, situating the Black community in the context of immigration is considered harmful by some, as it seems to continue to locate Black British people in the role of 'unwelcome guests'. It is also believed that the term 'immigrant' has become synonymous with inner-city problems (Knowles, 1990). The notion of the immigrant also seems to ignore the fact that most of the Black people now living in Britain were born here and look to no other place for a sense of belonging.

To make sense of the experience of a people, one needs to understand the circumstances under which they came to the host country, their sense of their own place in the scheme of things and to what extent successive generations share this view, have assimilated into the mainstream culture or have evolved different notions of their identity. The Black community consists of several generations, with varying degrees of assimilation into the majority culture with different expectations of the society.

Compared with the volume of work carried out on the epidemiology of psychosis in Caribbean people, there has been little interest in the themes of construction of the self in individuals from ethnic minorities, their understanding of illness, patterns of psychological adjustment, recourse to mental health agencies or, indeed, their attitude to professional medicine in general (Littlewood, 1993).

Perceptions in the Black media

Issues of identity, loss and other forms of suffering are not what has preoccupied the scientific or the popular press. The Black media currently focuses on two main issues related to psychiatry: misdiagnosis of schizophrenia (Chapter 6), widely reported in television documentaries; and deaths of African–Caribbean males in the care of psychiatric services. In general, the assumption is that there is something inherently racist in the practice of psychiatry and by implication that Blacks should avoid this institution. Accounts in the minority press (as Bahl has argued in Chapter 2) usually cover police involvement, compulsory admissions to forensic units, medication usually administered forcibly and in large quantities and the death of patients. However, key issues also include: (a) a lack of knowledge on the relatives' part of how to get access to care, hence compulsory admission; and (b) a failure in communication between relatives and hospital personnel when things go wrong.

Black people and psychiatry

There is now a well-recognised list of issues defining the relationship of Black people with mainstream psychiatry. It has been argued that while it is in the nature of psychiatry to have the power to exercise social control over individuals, social control is exercised over Black people to a disproportionate extent (Francis, 1989; Littlewood, 1993). This is expressed by greater use of compulsory admission procedures and greater use of secure facilities in the case of Black males (Littlewood, 1993; also see Chapter 6).

Once admitted, Black patients are more likely to be given physical treatment (that is, medication and electroconvulsive therapy; Mercer, 1984) rather than psychological treatment, more likely to be placed on depot medications and very unlikely to be offered psychotherapy. The interaction is that of a power struggle between the patient and the system, with coercion and containment being the outcome of the psychiatric system.

Recent work by Coker and colleagues in north London (see Chapter 4) speaks of secondary damage to the relationship between patients and psychiatric services. In that sample, access through primary care was higher than usually expected, but the negative perceptions of the patients occurred after they were engaged with the service.

A survey of patients in south-east London who had been targeted and responded positively to special outreach services because they were 'hard to engage' showed that they responded to approaches which were more flexible, less formal and hierarchical and which left them some measure of control over their lives. These patients had experienced previous dissatisfaction with the services, which centered a great deal around the power dynamic.

Black people in psychiatry

There are very few African and African–Caribbean doctors working in the National Health Service or in psychiatry. Black psychiatric nurses, who used to form a significant part of the staffing, are no longer present in large numbers in many institutions with predominantly Black patients. Nevertheless, the task of bringing an 'ethnic perspective' seems to fall on them. In this situation nurses often describe themselves as feeling 'de-skilled'. Within a team a Black nurse is regarded as having expertise mainly in the area of race and is seldom addressed on any other professional or technical issues in which she or he has competence or interest.

Given the hierarchical nature of most psychiatric teams the contribution made by nurses can be encouraged and valued or swept aside. When a person is consistently 'not heard' a feeling of being 'devalued' occurs and, eventually, only contributions which are felt to be safe are made. There is a tendency of the majority culture not to ask for clarification of a notion which seems different or strange but rather to position it in a familiar framework. It may be an attempt to understand the observation, but the value of the contribution of the Black team member is often lost in this situation. It becomes too difficult for them constantly to be burdened with an ethnic role within the context of their job.

It must not be forgotten that Black psychiatric workers at all levels experience racism on a daily basis in their own lives. Social workers and link-workers all report the same difficulties (Lloyd & Moodley, 1992). Reference has already been made to the isolation that Black workers may feel in their own communities for being a part of 'the system'; this isolation may be intensified at work if there are very few Black workers. It has to be understood that Black workers need to be part of the team, but also need to find mechanisms and support groups that help them to deal with the stress of their situation. Patients may expect a great deal from them, or if the patients are the victims of 'internalised racism' thay may expect nothing at all or may be hostile.

Resources in Black communities

A great deal of work is being done concerning the issue of mental illness in all communities, including predominantly Black communities. A survey in Southwark revealed that there were over 60 community organisations that were voluntary (Bhugra & La Grenade, 1997). The percentage of their clients with mental health needs ranged from 10 to 100%. Some of these organisations represented alternative forms of care to the formal sector, though many expressed that they would welcome increased collaboration with the formal sector. While they were aware of outreach community work by the formal sector they wanted more information on service provision. Many expressed an interest in increasing the dialogue with the formal sector and further information and training, particularly in the community care of people with mental illness (Bhugra & La Grenade, 1997). Data gathered from consultations around the UK (NHS Mental Health Task Force, 1994) show that organisations feel they could be more effective if there were regional organisations which could give their work greater recognition and greater voice (see Chapter 17).

The church is an important resource for many Black patients, and models of care utilising church-based initiatives have been tried and documented elsewhere. There is the notion that in the UK (NHS Mental Health Task Force, 1994) it is as yet an untapped resource, though in other cultures the church's function and value in Black mental health has been studied (Griffith *et al*, 1984).

Use of Black 'befrienders' and volunteers

The use of volunteers and 'befrienders' in psychiatry goes back to the 1970s. Training volunteers from particular ethnic communities seems to utilise the principle in a way that should benefit Black patients, the community and the mental health services. Training volunteers is a way of enhancing the resources of the Black community. The training begins with one section of the community involved in dialogue about the issues of mental illness and psychiatric practices, for example. This demystification of the subject should create a pool of potential allies for mental health services who might become important in the pathway into care.

Work in America (Neighbors *et al*, 1984) has demonstrated that in examining patterns of help-seeking behaviour in a community only 4.3% of individuals do so directly without informal consultation. Therefore, it would seem that volunteers represent an important possibility of increasing the dialogue between the services and the users. A volunteer who is well-matched to a patient's needs may function primarily as a befriender or as an advocate and the quality of the patient's life should be improved.

Currently, volunteers are affiliated mainly with the non-statutory sector, but there is a case for mental health teams to invest time in training and working with these individuals. Proper programme planning with mechanisms for selection, matching and supervision of volunteers is important if it is to be effective. Many professionals do not want to invest time in this way, and express the concern that a large volunteer programme will lower the standard of care by putting patients into the hands of non-professionals.

Government intiatives

Recommendations in respect of service delivery and mental health service development must include closer links between sectors, such as the social and health care services and the voluntary and public sector.

A good service

The World Health Organization has described the characteristics of a good primary health care service; the description seems no less applicable to mental health services for Black people. A good service should be: (a) available; (b) affordable; (c) accessible; (d) adaptable; (e) acceptable.

Although the first aspect is important, there is evidence that much of that which constitutes 'good practice' for ethnic minorities has been demonstrated on a small scale in Britain but is not widely available (see Chapter 22).

Access and acceptability seem to be linked. The primary care system in general assumes that Black people with mental distress have a mental illness, both because Black people do not feel welcome or understood by their general practitioner and also because there may be an inappropriate and exaggerated response to crises. It is not good enough to offer a service which seeks to offer the same package to everyone regardless of their needs. Even in conditions where medication is the main therapy, it is possible to exercise an 'ethnic sensitivity', for example, in the approaches offered to the family, the type of occupational therapy activities envisaged, the willingness to engage themes like racism and concerns about family in the patient's treatment package.

A good community service should encourage a variety of approaches and responses which the patient can have access to. There may be counselling offered by a voluntary service operating from an ethnocentric point of view, as well as non-governmental organisations offering services targeted to women or particular problems. An important principle often forgotten is that the service user should be consulted about the choices as far as possible.

Principles

(a) The service should be 'colour-sensitive' not 'colour-blind'. Services are often offered to individuals irrespective of their needs, and the packages inevitably reflect the perceptions of the majority culture of what is appropriate, and therefore may not be acceptable to Black service users.

(b) The services should emphasise care and collaboration with the community, rather than control and containment.

(c) Services should cooperate with the community, recognising that currently, Black communities have an inherent mistrust of the formal mental health care system. Working with the Black media and developing a policy within the system for dealing with media is critical. Often the media want information on specific issues and are not able to speak with anyone. This simply reinforces the notion that things are being hidden.

Other approaches to working with the community

Working with non-governmental organisations

This may involve extensive input of time in becoming familiar with organisations that exist, finding out about their activities, what their needs are and what their prime focus is. Clear communication about service location, how they can be accessed and, where relevant, who the link-workers are, must be conveyed.

Recognising the role of the church in the community's life

These include mainstream churches with large Black populations as well as the usually smaller 'Black churches'. This is a difficult area as the mental health services are sometimes seen as being in opposition to religion.

Inviting the community to become part of the planning process

There are many pitfalls in this approach including the reality that the most active people in 'community participation' are often not really representative and may be following a different agenda. Consultation is still possible and true knowledge of a community gradually makes the process easier.

Staffing should reflect the ethnicity of the service users

Mental health professionals have always had to work across ethnic 'boundaries' and matching patients strictly according to ethnicity is not always desirable or practical. However, many of the difficulties of communication and culture can be more easily dealt with if there are Black staff involved in the planning and running of the service.

The range of services should reflect the community requirements

The regional task force seminars singled out services they considered to be important. These included: (a) crises services; (b) 24-hour and weekend services; (c) women-only services; (d) appropriate counselling.

Reference has already been made to the failure of Black people to access the 'communication therapies'. Many of the voluntary organisations (Fanon, African–Caribbean Mental Health Association, Isis) offer these services within the limits of their staff. It is important that mainstream services either purchase services from these organisations or develop their own capacity to deliver them.

References

BARKER, P. (1973) Problems of migrants. In *Basic Child Psychiatry*, pp. 159–162. London: Crosby Lockwood Staples.

BHAT, A., BURKE, A. W. & FALKOWSKI, W. (1984) Psychiatric workers as emotional beings: The emotional reactions of staff following the Brixton riots. *International Journal of Social Psychiatry*, **30**, 9–15.

BHUGRA, D. & LA GRENADE, J. (1997) Community organisations' expectations of mental health statutory services. *Irish Journal of Psychological Medicine*, **14**, 57–59.

COCHRANE, R. (1979) Psychological and behavioural disturbance in West Indians, Indians and Pakistanis in Britain: a comparison of rates among children and adults. *British Journal of Psychiatry,* **134,** 201–210.

FRANCIS, E. (1989) Black people, 'dangerousness' and psychiatric compulsion. In *Mental Health Care in Crisis* (eds A. Bracx & C. Grimshaw). London: Pluto.

GRIFFITH, E. E. H., YOUNG, J. H. & SMITH, D. H. (1984) An analysis of the therapeutic elements in a Black church service. *Hospital and Community Psychiatry,* **35,** 464–469.

KNOWLES, C. (1990) Afro-Caribbeans and schizophrenia: How does psychiatry deal with issues of race, culture and ethnicity. *Journal of Social Policy,* **20,** 191–213.

LITTLEWOOD, R. (1993) Ideology, camouflage or contingency? Racism in British psychiatry. *Transcultural Psychiatry Research Review,* **30,** 243–290.

MERCER, K. (1984) Black communities' experience of psychiatric services. *International Journal of Social Psychiatry,* **30,** 22–27.

LLOYD, K. & MOODLEY, P. (1992) Psychotropic medication and ethnicity: an in-patient survey. *Social Psychiatry and Psychiatric Epidemiology,* **27,** 95–101.

NHS MENTAL HEALTH TASK FORCE (1994) *Black Mental Health – A Dialogue for Change.* Leeds: NHS Executive.

NEIGHBORS, H. W. & JACKSON, J. S. (1984) The use of informal and formal help: Four patterns of illness behaviour in the Black Community. *American Journal of Community Psychology,* **12,** 29–44.

19 Role of the general practitioner in the management of mental illness in ethnic minorities

SANGEETA PATEL

The 5.9% of the population of England that described their ethnic origin as other than White in the 1991 census are distributed unevenly around the country with a predominance in certain areas within inner cities (Balarajan & Raleigh, 1992). The general practioners (GPs) within those areas will have greater proportions of patients from Black and minority ethnic groups registered with them (Gillam *et al*, 1989). Those from minority ethnic groups have been reported to consult their GP more frequently than the White population (Gillam *et al*, 1989).

GPs are often the first point of call to people requiring health care and have the potential to establish long-term relationships with individual patients. They commonly have access to their past medical records and knowledge of their social and family circumstances and are therefore well placed to assess the mental health status of their patients. Management of psychological morbidity can place a huge demand upon GPs who can only be effective with adequate secondary support.

Primary prevention of mental illness in ethnic minorities

Primary prevention of mental illness in general practice involves the identification and modification of known risk factors. Although these may be dependent upon much wider changes in society and its values, the GP, if he or she is aware of some of the effects of these, can often intervene and modify them (Harris, 1996). The GP will often know which patient groups are faced with unemployment, poverty and overcrowding: all of these are more likely to affect ethnic minorities (Brown, 1984; Rudat, 1994*a*). The GP may also be aware of individual stressful life-events, such as marital breakdown, bereavement or physical illness (Harris, 1996). He or she can often modify some of the effects of these, such as providing certificates for absence from work, supporting applications for alternative housing or benefits for caring for disabled dependents. The GP can make those from different ethnic groups aware of the benefits to which they may be entitled or direct them to other sources of advice.

Secondary prevention

Secondary prevention of mental illness in general practice involves screening, early detection of symptoms and treatment. This relies upon good access to the primary care team as well as effective early diagnosis of mental illness by the GP.

Access to general practice

All residents of the UK, the European Community and those from countries who have a reciprocal arrangement with Britain are entitled to register with a GP and receive health care free at the point of delivery for illnesses that develop while they are in the UK. For other patients or those with pre-existing illnesses the GP is entitled to charge; the cost is at their discretion.

Ninety-eight per cent of people are registered with a GP; unlike many other registers, those from ethnic minority groups are not significantly under-represented (Balajaran *et al*, 1989; Rudat, 1994*b*). The choice of GP may be limited for those patients for whom the origin of the GP or the languages they speak is paramount (Pharoah, 1995). Indeed, a higher proportion of Asian patients are registered with Asian GPs (Balajaran *et al*, 1989; Rudat, 1994*b*; Pharoah, 1995).

On average, 70% of people see their GP within one year. Other members of the primary health care team are in contact with some particularly high-risk groups: families with young children are seen by health visitors, the housebound elderly (over 75 years old) are offered visits by practice nurses, the disabled requiring nursing care are seen by district nurses, etc.

GPs do not routinely systematically screen for mental illness, but because of their exposure to a large proportion of their patients they are able to screen opportunistically those patients that they believe are at high risk and those who present to the GP with early symptoms of mental illness.

Filters to psychiatric care

Relationship of annual period prevalence of mental disorders

As has already been discussed in Chapter 4, Goldberg & Huxley (1992) described the filters to psychiatric care, displayed in Fig. 1. Per year, of the population at risk, 71% consult their GP (circle A), 31.5% have a distressing episode of psychological symptoms lasting at least one week during the year (circle B – the overlap of circles A and B represents those who consult their GP). The GP diagnoses 10.5% as having a definite mental disorder (circle C) and 2.35% are referred to specialist mental health services during the year (circle D).

Clearly these filters are not always in the best interests of users of mental health services and attempts have been made to break down barriers to further care in the majority culture with health education messages, such as the 'Defeat Depression' campaign to make the public aware of the importance of presentation of psychological symptoms to members of the primary health care team (Priest, 1991). As with so much health education propaganda, it is least available to those who may need it most – such as those of low socio-economic status and those in ethnic minority groups.

Balajaran *et al* (1989) reported data from the General Household Surveys and found that consultation rates with GPs varied among different ethnic groups when adjusted for age and socio-demographic factors. Indian, Pakistani and West Indian people had

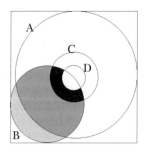

Fig. 1

Venn diagram showing the relationship of disorders at Levels 1, 2, 3 and 4 (after Goldberg & Huxley, 1992). The square represents the population at risk: A, people who consulted their doctor during the period of a year; B, people who experienced an episode of psychological distress during the year (Level 1); C, people identified by their doctor as being mentally ill (Level 3); D, people referred to mental health services (Level 4);☐, did not pass through first filter (i.e. were ill but did not consult); ■, did not pass through second filter (i.e. their illness was not recognised by the doctor); ■,did not pass through third filter (i.e. were not referred to mental health services) higher consultation rates. This finding was repeated in the Health Education Authority survey of 3500 adults; significantly higher GP consultation rates were found among African–Caribbean and south Asian people (Rudat, 1994*b*). In Fig. 1, circle A would be larger for these groups of people. The overlap of circle A with circle B represents those who present their psychological distress to their GP. Gillam *et al* (1989), in a study of a large urban practice over a two-year period, reported that consultation rates with GPs for mental disorders in southern Irish, West Indian and Asian people were lower than that for native British people. However, this may have been a reflection of a difference or inadequacy in the categories used by the GPs for these ethnic groups or an actual difference in morbidity. Assessment of psychological morbidity data needs to take account of the applicability of Western criteria upon those of different ethnic origins (Kleinman, 1987; Bracken 1993). The correct identification of mental disorders by GPs (circle C) and their referral to mental health services (circle D) are affected by race and culture at all levels.

Diagnosis by GPs of mental illness in people from ethnic minorities

As generalists, GPs must have a wide, but not necessarily detailed, knowledge of illnesses prevalent among their patients. Consequently GPs are more often aware of the central themes of psychiatric research than they are of its limitations. Most psychiatric research about people of Black and other minority ethnic groups has involved hospitalised patients and has concentrated upon the differences between them and native British communities. This has tended to reflect popular stereotypes, such as that of Black people being more prone to schizophrenia or cannabis psychosis, that of reluctance to be referred to psychiatric hospital, specifically among Asian people (lest it affect marriage prospects), and that of Asian and African–Caribbean people presenting mental illness somatically (Fernando, 1991).

GPs are often able to cover only limited psychological ground in their short consultations, particularly in the presence of physical symptoms and communication difficulties: the pressure to establish a working diagnosis will mean that they will tend to focus upon those which they believe to be most likely. Psychiatric diagnoses by GPs are therefore more likely to reflect medical and popular stereotypes (Fernando, 1991). People from ethnic minorities have been reported to be more likely to present their psychological symptoms somatically (Kirmayer, 1984; Mumford, 1992; Krause, 1994). GPs may not be clear regarding the degree of physical and psychological components of the illness and may perform physical investigations unnecessarily or reluctantly. Negative stereotypes of ethnic minorities abound inside and outside the medical profession (Townsend, 1979; Gilman, 1990). GPs and other health care workers have been reported to hold less positive views towards their Asian patients than their White patients (Ahmad *et al*, 1991; Bowler, 1993). Nevertheless, GPs, as they work intimately with individual patients, constantly have their stereotypes challenged and many will come to accept that generalisations do not always apply to individuals.

If verbal communication is hindered by language difficulties, then assessment of mental health will be very limited. However, the emphasis upon language as the chief inhibitor to communication has been criticised (Bowes & Domokos, 1995; Patel, 1995). The percentage of people who do not speak English is decreasing: in 1994, the rate among Indians was found to be 15% (8% of men), among Pakistanis 28% and among the Bangladeshi community 41% (Rudat, 1994*a*). Generally, language problems tend to be dealt with *ad hoc* using family members, friends and neighbours or another worker on-site who speaks the same language (Pharoah, 1995). These strategies are rarely appropriate because of issues of confidentiality, the shift in the balance of power between patient and their translator, who may be a family member, and the tendency of the untrained to interpret rather than just translate (Pharoah, 1995). Patients and GPs need access to suitable interpreting and advocacy services, particularly in areas with a large proportion of any minority ethnic group who are not fluent in English.

GPs have been reported to fail to make a diagnosis of depression in half of their patients (Freeling *et al*, 1985; Tylee & Freeling, 1989) but this figure is less for Asian females (Jacob *et al*, 1998). The presence of concurrent physical illness or initial presentation of physical symptoms, both of which are more likely in Black and minority ethnic communities, has been reported to make it less likely for the GP to diagnose depression (Tylee & Freeling, 1989). GPs with less knowledge or consideration of depressive illness in consultations or those who have not elicited the cues pointing towards depression have also been reported to be less likely to make the diagnosis (Tylee & Freeling, 1989): those GPs with high proportions of patients from ethnic minorities are often those working with the least resources, for whom it is more difficult to obtain training in mental illness management (Pharoah, 1995). Doctors have more difficulty in assessing the contribution of cultural factors in patients from cultures different from their own (Helman, 1990).

Early treatment of mental illness in ethnic minorities in general practice

There is a trend towards the management of minor psychiatric morbidity in primary care. GPs have more access to counsellors working in the primary care setting and are exposed to education, such as the Defeat Depression campaign, encouraging them to manage more psychological illness in primary care (Pharoah, 1995). GPs have been reported to refer fewer of their patients from Black and other minority ethnic groups (than their White patients) to allied members of the community team (Pharoah, 1995). Multilingual link-workers have been reported to see their own role to include counselling, but only a small proportion of their patients are referred from GPs (Priest, 1991).

Patients from Black and other ethnic minority communities are rarely referred for psychotherapy (Kareem & Littlewood, 1992; Lipsedge, 1993). This may be because of the assumption that they lack the psychological mindedness, verbal sophistication or capacity for insight (Kareem & Littlewood, 1992; Lipsedge, 1993). Racially sensitive psychotherapy has been reported to be effective (Moorhouse, 1992). Even when such facilities are available, GPs are not always aware of them (Pharoah, 1995).

Tertiary prevention

Tertiary prevention of mental illness involves the assessment and treatment of acute and chronic illness and monitoring to prevent recurrences. Unfortunately, it is still often the case that GPs are only involved with the care of their mentally ill patients from ethnic minorities when they become acutely ill and require referral to hospital.

Referral to hospital by GPs

Referral is a complex process influenced by the views of both the patient and doctor (Morgan, 1989). Black people are less likely to be referred for further psychiatric or psychological treatment (Kareem & Littlewood, 1992; Lipsedge, 1993). African–Caribbean people are less likely to be referred because of a mental illness by their GP at the early stage of the illness (Owens *et al*, 1991; also see Chapter 7) and are more likely to be admitted to hospital by the police or social services under a section of the Mental Health Act (Moodley & Perkins, 1991). Referral is a complex process influenced by views of both patient and doctor. Gillam *et al* (1989) reported lower consultation rates with GPs for mental disorders in southern Irish, West Indian and Asian people than native British people. GPs may not attend to early illness among their Black and ethnic minority patients either because they fail to recognise the symptoms of mental illness, fail to ascribe them to psychiatric illness, recognise but do not refer them because of actual or ascribed stigma among these minority communities, are ignorant about the importance of early treatment or do not have access to suitable local services. Education of the public and GPs has in the past only been aimed towards English speakers and, although it has recently begun to address the needs of ethnic minority groups, much more is called for.

Follow-up

The GP will often have access to the family or local support networks of those with mental illness and can involve them in the care and monitoring of the patients themselves, both during the illness and afterwards to prevent recurrences. The continuity of care by a single GP, who, even if they were not involved in the initial presentation of the illness, should at least have been informed, will often enable him or her to be especially aware of the early signs of relapse in individual patients. The GP is the first point of call for physical as well as mental problems and can monitor for recurrences opportunistically, when systematic monitoring fails. Patients with schizophrenia have been reported to be more likely to have seen their GP than their psychiatrist after discharge from hospital (Pantelis *et al*, 1988; Melzer *et al*, 1991).

GPs themselves require appropriate support in the management of their ethnic minority patients who have suffered acute mental illnesses or continue to suffer with chronic mental illness. This support includes education for specific features of recurrences, treatment options available and clear information and access to local facilities.

Recent strategic changes and opportunities

There has been much strategic change in primary care over the past three years. In broad terms this has led to more local responsibility for primary care provision, which should be more appropriate for and accountable to the local population. More specifically, primary care groups and primary care pilot schemes consisting of a conglomeration of primary care teams serving around 100 000 patients each have been set up. These will work with health authorities, community trusts and local authorities to commission health care and develop and implement local 'Health Improvement Programmes'. They will have the power and local flexibility to negotiate services appropriate for their patients, which can thus specifically benefit ethnic minority communities with high proportions in particular areas. Furthermore, these bodies will be publicly accountable and subject to quality standards developed locally and nationally. A new 'National Performance Network' will focus upon six areas of performance, one of which is fair access to services for patients of all social and ethnic groups. The primary care groups or pilot project schemes thus have the scope to provide specific services for ethnic minority groups, such as interpreting and advocacy services, culturally appropriate counselling or psychotherapy and training in cultural awareness for members of the primary care team.

There have also been key changes in medical education over recent years. The undergraduate curriculum has changed to provide a limited 'core curriculum' which is compulsory for all students and 'special study modules' for selected students. Within the core curriculum, themes that span across cultures are encouraged and the special study modules afford an opportunity to teach on specific cultural or ethnic themes. Both undergraduate and postgraduate teaching are increasingly being conducted in the community (for example some pre-registration house officer posts are been undertaken in general practice). Cross-cultural awareness training and education is increasingly being supported in primary care (for example, the Royal College of General Practitioners recently commissioned a programme for cultural awareness for GP registrars).

There are many opportunities for improving the mental health care for ethnic minorities provided by GPs, although, in times of change, the needs of 'minority' groups are often marginalised. It will require those with energy, commitment and an understanding of the complexities of provision of cross-cultural primary health care to use these opportunities. In this chapter, I have tried to outline the role and perspectives of the GPs in negotiating the complex issues which determine their management of mental illness in ethnic minorities.

References

Ahmad, W. I. U., Baker, M. & Kemohan, E. M. (1991) General practitioners' perceptions of Asian and non-Asian patients. *Family Practice*, **8**, 52–56.

Balarajan, R., Yuen, P. & Raleigh, V. S. (1989) Ethnic differences in General Practice Consultations. *British Medical Journal*, **299**, 958–960.

—— & RALEIGH, V. S. (1992) The ethnic population of England and Wales: the 1991 census. *Health Trends*, **24**, 113–116.

BOWES, A. M. & DOMOKOS, T. M. (1995) South Asian women and their GPs: some issues of communication. *Social Science and Health*, **1**, 22–33.

BOWLER, I. (1993) 'They're not the same as us': midwives' stereotypes of South Asian descent maternity patients. *Social Health and Illness*, **15**, 157–178.

BRACKEN, P. (1993) Post-empiricism and psychiatry: meaning and methodology in cross-cultural research. *Social Science and Medicine*, **36**, 265–272.

BROWN, C. (1984) *Black and White Britain: the Third PSI Survey.* London: Heinemann.

FERNANDO, S. (1991) Applied psychiatry. In *Mental Health, Race and Culture* (ed. S. Fernando), pp. 113–145. London: Macmillan.

FREELING, P., RAO, B. M., PAYKEL, E. S., *et al* (1985) Unrecognised depression in general practice. *British Medical Journal*, **290**, 1880–1883.

GILLAM, S. J., JARMAN, B., WHITE, P., *et al* (1989) Ethnic differences in consultation rates in urban general practice. *British Medical Journal*, **299**, 953–957.

GILMAN, S. (1990) Introduction: What are stereotypes and why use texts to study them? In *Difference and Pathology: Stereotypes of Sexuality, Race and Madness* (ed. S. Gilman), pp. 15–35. London: Cornell University Press.

GOLDBERG, D. & HUXLEY, P. (1992) Models for mental illness. In *Common Mental Disorders. A Bio-Social Model* (eds D. Goldberg & P. Huxley), pp. 1–14, 30–52. London: Routledge.

HARRIS, T. (1996) Primary prevention: assessing the relevance of life-events and difficulties among primary care attenders. In *The Prevention of Mental Illness in Primary Care* (eds T. Kendrick, A. Tylee & P. Freeling), pp.41–56. Cambridge: Cambridge University Press.

HELMAN, C. (1990) Cross-cultural psychiatry. In *Culture, Health and Illness* (ed. C. Helman), pp. 214–248. Bristol: Wright.

JACOB, K. S., BHUGRA, D., LLOYD, K., *et al* (1998) Common mental disorders, explanatory models and consultation behaviour in Indian women living in the UK. *Journal of the Royal Society of Medicine*, **91**, 66–71.

KAREEM, J. & LITTLEWOOD, R. (1992) *Intercultural Therapy: Themes, Interpretations and Practice.* Oxford: Blackwell.

KIRMAYER, L. (1984) Culture, affect and somatisation. *Transcultural Psychiatric Research Review*, **21**, 159–188.

KLEINMAN, A. (1987) Anthropology and psychiatry: the role of culture in cross-cultural research on illness. *British Journal of Psychiatry*, **151**, 447–454.

KRAUSE, I. B. (1994) Numbers and meaning: a dialogue in cross-cultural psychiatry. *Journal of the Royal Society of Medicine*, **87**, 278–282.

LIPSEDGE, M. (1993) Mental health: access to care for Black and ethnic minority people. In *Access to Health Care for People from Black and Ethnic Minorities* (eds A. Hopkins & V. Bahl), pp. 169–185. London: Royal College of Physicians.

MELZER, D., HALE, A. S., MALIK, S. J., *et al* (1991) Community care for patients with schizophrenia one year after hospital discharge. *British Medical Journal*, **303**, 1023 –1026.

MOODLEY, P. & PERKINS, R. (1991) Routes to psychiatric in-patient care in an inner-London borough. *Social Psychiatry and Psychiatric Epidemiology*, **26**, 47–51.

MOORHOUSE, S. (1992) Quantitative research in intercultural therapy. In *Intercultural Therapy* (eds J. Kareem & R. Littlewood), pp. 83–98. Oxford: Blackwell.

MORGAN, D. (1989) Psychiatric cases: an ethnography of the referral process. *Psychological Medicine*, **19**, 743–753.

MUMFORD, D. (1992) Detection of psychiatric disorders among Asian patients presenting with somatic symptoms. *British Journal of Hospital Medicine*, **147**, 202–204.

OWENS, D., HARRISON, G. & BOOT, D. (1991) Ethnic factors in voluntary and compulsory admissions. *Psychological Medicine*, **21**, 185–196.

PANTELIS, C., TAYLOR, J. & CAMPBELL, P. (1988) The South Camden Schizophrenia Survey: an experience of community-based research. *Psychiatric Bulletin*, **12**, 98–101.

PATEL, S. (1995) Language is not the only barrier. *British Medical Journal,* **310,**194.

PHAROAH, C. (1995) *Primary Health Care for Elderly People from Black and Minority Ethnic Communities.* London: HMSO.

PRIEST, R. G. (1991) A new initiative on depression. *British Journal of General Practioners,* **41,** 487.

RUDAT, K. (1994*a*) Demographic features. In *Black and Minority Ethnic Groups in England, Health and Lifestyles,* pp. 22–40. London: Health Education Authority Publications.

—— (1994*b*) Use of health services. In *Black and Minority Ethnic Groups in England, Health and Lifestyles,* pp. 54–78. London: Health Education Authority Publications.

TOWNSEND, J. M. (1979) Stereotypes and mental illness: a comparison with ethnic stereotypes. *Culture, Medicine and Psychiatry,* **3,** 205–230.

TYLEE, A., & FREELING, P. (1989) The recognition, diagnosis and acknowledgment of depressive disorders by general practitioners. In *Depression: An Integrative Approach* (eds E. Paykel & K. Herbst), pp. 216–232. London: Heinemann.

20 Voluntary organisations' perspective on mental health needs

PAT GRAY

Controversies about the existence and aetiology of mental illness in Britain's Black population continue to be ardently debated (see discussions in Chapters 2–6). This has been referred to by Francis *et al* (1989) as a "major crisis" in psychiatry in relation to race, notably the disproportionately high rates of some types of mental illness among African–Caribbeans. The increase in attempted suicide and self-poisoning by Asian women in recent years has added to that debate (see Chapter 12). There is a wealth of empirical evidence which shows that Britain's Black population has a different experience of health and welfare services compared with White people. There is a particular sense of disadvantage in relation to services. It is this disparity in experiences that has been the motivational force for the Black community to seek alternatives to institutional psychiatry and which has given rise to a growth of Black community mental health agencies in the voluntary sector.

Issues

For many years the Black community has been making critical observations of psychiatry (see Chapter 18). One of the biggest problems in psychiatry is the lack of adequate care given to the Black communities. There is a lack of research into the views of users, but key themes to emerge from conferences and public meetings are as follows:

  (a) dissatisfaction with services;
  (b) lack of satisfaction with the treatment currently being provided;

(c) there are only limited alternatives to physical treatments;
(d) a feeling of being misunderstood and views are not respected;
(e) information is not shared;
(f) cultural and spiritual needs are not adequately met;
(g) there are language barriers;
(h) like the majority community, ethnic minority groups would like to have more say in their treatment and planning of services.

Constant concerns voiced repeatedly by the users of the service (patients), relatives, carers, those working within the field and campaigning organisations such as the African–Carribbean Mental Health Association (ACMHA; based in London) and MIND serve as an indictment of psychiatry. Furthermore, it has led to the Black community becoming increasingly frustrated with present-day psychiatry and allied disciplines (see Chapter 15).

There appears to be poor appreciation of the inter-relationship between ethnicity, race, culture and mental health and the social, political and economic status of Britain's Black communities. These determine the level of response and provision of resources to the health care needs of Black communities; however, historically they have resulted in unequal access to service provision. The findings continue to fuel the debate about the racism and Eurocentrism that underpins British psychiatry. Smaje (1995) suggests that three main points underlie the findings:

(a) psychiatrists may be prone to invoking racial stereotypes when making diagnoses;
(b) psychiatrists may mistake minor symptoms or people's belief systems because of their lack of awareness of ethnic and cultural differences;
(c) psychiatry is seen as an instrument of social control.

Role of psychiatry

In its endeavour to establish itself as a discipline, psychiatry has historically gleaned its knowledge from various theories and research which could be challenged for their racist ideologies (Fernando, 1988). As a body of knowledge, psychiatry is seen to rely heavily on its research which it presents as a knowledge of truth in its argument for the monopoly in the field of mental health. The subjects of research are always the 'other' group, and are seen as different, inferior, less civilised, interesting, a problem and, more importantly, unequal. For a long time Black people have been the preoccupation of 'White gaze' in various fields of research in an attempt to define Black culture and groups, the Black family, Black behaviour and the Black psyche. The tools used have been from a White perspective and repertoire, which are most fitting for White, Western people – not for Black people living in a Western context (see Chapters 4, 5 and 6). In so doing, Black people continue to be pathologised on the basis of their difference, thereby adding to a defeat resulting in a dependency on White, Eurocentric values and attitudes.

Gaze on psychiatry

It would seem appropriate for the gaze to be shifted to psychiatry, in order to address the racism that exists within psychiatry. There needs to be urgent, fundamental change within the discipline of psychiatry, which will not only involve a re-examination of the basic concepts of psychiatric theory and practice, but will also challenge the Eurocentric ideologies on which it is based. As an institution that exists in a racist society it also has not managed to escape the impact of racism.

Psychiatry, as a discipline, ought to address some of the following questions:

(a) How have various ideologies in psychiatry influenced its thinking about Black groups who do not have the same amount of power that psychiatry has?
(b) Has psychiatry considered what the existence of racism in society and its role has encouraged or allowed it to do to less powerful groups?
(c) How does the power that psychiatry is perceived to have and the impact of disadvantage perceived by Black people discourage psychiatry from responding to the needs of Black and minority ethnic groups?

Psychiatry cannot escape the legacy of colonialism and paternalism that forms the backdrop of its relationship with the Black community. The creative abilities of psychiatry to diagnose past illnesses such as drapetomania (diagnosed in slaves who ran away from their plantations) and in more recent times Ganja (cannabis) psychoses have only served to mask its continual confusion and failure in appropriately addressing the needs of Black people.

While Black communities recognise that the problem is not with the Black community, but rather with the structure of psychiatry, psychiatry's perceptions of Black people vary.

Health service needs

The NHS Mental Health Task Force (1994) completed its extensive cross-country survey on race, mental health and community services in 1995. It met with various mental health agencies and found:

(a) Despite the ongoing dialogue over the years between local organisations and statutory services, research evidence and recommendations for change, there are still few facilities that cater for the needs of Black communities.

(b) Where services do exist for Black people they are usually set up and organised by Black people themselves in reaction to the lack of attention paid by statutory services to the needs of communities.

(c) Experiences of users and the Black communities were negative.

(d) Gaps still remain in the service.

(e) Consultation continues to be poor and needs to be more effective; users and the Black community want a greater say and role in the planning of services.

For at least three decades within the field of psychiatry there has been an ongoing debate about the lack of adequate provision for Black communities, about the racism that exists within its structure, and about poor user involvement (see Chapter 17).

Given the evidence that we have about the high admission rates for Black groups, it is striking that Black people are still under-represented as employees at all levels within psychiatry. Why does psychiatry and other related disciplines find it so difficult to recruit Black staff and address this crisis? Fernando (1988) asserts that there are various devices such as institutional racism, language and preferment to Eurocentric ideologies that are used by psychiatry and allied professions to maintain a White institution. If this is the case, the implications for Black staff working within predominantly White institutions are not dissimilar to those for Black communities trying to survive in a White majority society (see Chapter 18).

Voluntary sector

What does the Black voluntary sector have to offer that is different from existing services? We have to consider the context from which voluntary services emerge and how they are constructed. Prior to being established there is usually a history of ongoing debate among community and professional workers and, in some cases, carers or campaigners. For example, the African–

Carribbean Mental Health Project (ACMHP; Manchester) was set up by community workers and Black and White professionals, but not before years of discussion, a working party and two public meetings. The Project came out of the belief and concern that present services were inaccessible, inappropriate and insensitive to the needs of the local African–Caribbean community. Most of the users of Black mental health projects and other minority group organisations that exist across the country have a history of being misunderstood, misdiagnosed, hospitalised and have experienced a lack of alternative treatments such as counselling or psychotherapy, and the excessive use of drugs. Over the past few years Asian mental health projects have also been established on the basis of unmet need due to cultural differences, language barriers and religious beliefs.

The Black voluntary sector, in recognising these differences and misunderstandings, offers a unique service to the Black community. It is a service that is underpinned by a perspective which cannot be matched by present-day mainstream psychiatric services. This Black or Afrocentric perspective is fundamental to the existence and provision of care to the Black community. It is the basis for understanding the political reality of Black people's experiences, the hardships and racism that they endure, and is therefore appropriate for their cultural and racial identity needs. Unlike mainstream models it is not symptom-focused but deals with the whole person, offering both specialised and generic input.

Traditionally arising from some form of community action, these organisations are well-placed to develop innovative styles of practice that meet the culturally diverse needs of its community. Their main aim is to provide appropriate forms of care and support to users of the service, relatives and carers. They are able to access networks on behalf of the service user, which statutory services find difficult. In addition to this, many organisations are seeking ways to challenge the existing racial inequalities and the lack of appropriate care that exist with mainstream services, but more pertinently the fundamental body of knowledge that underpins psychiatry and allied disciplines. These services are generally trusted and supported by the community but face one great threat – the lack of appropriate and guaranteed funding. Most of these groups are awarded time-limited funding contracts or insubstantial funding for the adequate employment of skilled staff with which to meet the demands of both community and statutory services. They also live with the continuous threat of having the funds cut, significantly enough to threaten the stability and life of the service.

Role of the Department of Health

The Community Care Act 1990 and the Department of Health (1993) guidelines for meeting the Health of the Nation targets emphasise the problem of the unmet mental health needs of Britain's Black communities. Both the Act and the guidelines make it clear that services need to be enhanced to provide culturally appropriate facilities. The directives came at a time when the opportunity for fundamental change in the relationship between statutory agencies and the voluntary sector could take place. However, this has been thwarted by the argument that 'needs outweigh resources' as services are expected to provide culturally appropriate facilities at a time when financial constraints exist and there is no statutory requirement to ensure that the mental health needs of the Black communities are being provided for. As Bahl states (Chapter 2), with the change in government, priorities have changed and are aimed at tackling social exclusion. Despite these social, political and economic factors the work that voluntary organisations do is commendable, often going unrecognised by mainstream funding bodies, especially in long-term planning strategies. Health authorities, trusts and local authorities have a tremendous influence on determining the

TABLE 1
Black voluntary mental health sector v.statutory psychiatric services

Set up by Black community and professionals	Set up by White professionals
User involvement	Little user involvement
Alternative models that are Afrocentric/culture specific	Eurocentric models dominate the service
Strength model	Weakness model
Appropriate, accessible, sensitive	Inappropriate, inaccessible to needs, insensitive to needs
Lack of recognition	Recognition
Expertise in Black people's experiences	Little expertise in Black people's experiences
Offers choice	Offers little choice
Recognises diversity in the Black community	Undifferentiated view of Black people
Acknowledges racism and other social factors	Impact of racism/social factors often ignored
Poorly resourced	Well resourced
Non-racist ideology	Racist ideology
Advocacy	No true advocacy
Models of good practice	Models of good practice?

budget, prioritising services, purchasing contracts and determining strategies, yet continually exclude the participation and the voice of the Black communities in the decision-making process.

A brief overview of some of the main differences between the Black voluntary mental health sector and statutory psychiatric services is shown in Table 1. These differences form the basis of the underlying argument for the Black voluntary sector to keep its services separate from mainstream psychiatry. This presents something of a double-bind for Black services, as mainstream services are reluctant to support Black groups and give them responsibility for services, however, psychiatry may then itself fail to address adequately the service needs of Black communities through its own mainstream provision. Therefore, the Black mental health organisations that exist do so because needs are continually being unmet by the statutory services. It is on the basis of this rationale that they are necessary for the mental health and well-being of the Black community.

Separate or together

The argument for separation of services is one which creates varied responses from funders. For example, some statutory services will fund a local Black organisation as a way of dealing with their obligations to the local community. The inherent danger here is that the Black organisation is left to become overwhelmed by the demands from the community and other services. In the process of funding the Black organisation, the statutory services remain unchanged and do not truly address their own failure of responsibility in relation to the provision of appropriate care to the Black community. The argument for Black mental health agencies to remain separate is based on the importance of preserving what makes the service successful, that is, its sense of Black identity and values, accessibility and creativity in its work with the Black community. Integration into mainstream services in its current form would directly threaten these qualities.

Accountability

Accountability in the services is more than an accountability process for services. McLean (1994) offers a practical way forward with the concept that structured power differences are central to our society and they need to be recognised and addressed in order that the groups which have been marginalised and oppressed can have their voices heard. It is important to recognise that this concept of accountability is primarily concerned with addressing injustice, as McLean goes on to assert:

> "it provides members of the dominant group (psychiatry) with the information necessary for them to stand against the oppressive practices implicit within their own culture of which they will be totally unaware".

Could psychiatry consider what the benefits might be for itself in transforming its practice in this way? Also, what might the benefits be to Britain's Black communities?

The concept of accountability can be addressed by recognising the reality of the power that it has and how it is exerted on an individual level as well as a hierarchical level. Structured power differences already exist in relation to race, gender, class, sexuality, ethnicity and mobility in our society, as well as other social factors such as housing, employment and health care. For Britain's Black population it is through these differences that they experience the social injustice of discrimination that they speak out about. McLean's notion of accountability is based upon "the recognition that the best judges of when an injustice has occurred are those who have experienced it".

For members of psychiatry and allied psychiatric services to participate in this process of accountability a clear commitment is required to do whatever is necessary in order to understand the perspectives of Black people and their experiences of psychiatry.

Recommendations

Some key issues need to be highlighted for the providers and purchasers. These are:

(a) Assessment, diagnosis and treatment – which should be culturally sensitive
(b) Funding – which needs to be substantive and long-term.
(c) Research – of Black service users' views.
(d) Consultation – involving Black service users when planning services.
(e) Accountability of psychiatric services to the Black communities.
(f) Alternative models should be used that are Afrocentric-based.
(g) Power and control issues – the balance needs to be redressed.
(h) Employment opportunities for those with mental health problems.

(i)   Family involvement in the planning of care programmes.
(j)   Support for carers/relatives.
(k) The need for Black advocacy.
(l)   Community education.
(m) Housing – proper supported housing is required.
(n) Criminal justice system needs to address Black mental health issues.

This chapter has offered an insight into some of the key issues that Black and ethnic minority groups face when they seek help from statutory services when they suffer from mental ill health. Services need to develop in a culturally sensitive manner, making it clear that all members of the local population have equal access to them. There should be discussions with purchasers about the appropriate services that will be offered. Voluntary organisations have a key role to play and can give insightful perspectives into the needs of Black and ethnic minority groups and can also succeed in improving compliance and meeting holistic approaches to mental health.

Acknowledgements

I thank the members of the African Mental Health Project (Manchester), their families and carers.

References

DEPARTMENT OF HEALTH (1993) *Health of the Nation.* London: HMSO.
FERNANDO, S. (1988) *Race and Culture in Psychiatry.* London: Croom Helm.
FRANCIS, E., DAVID, J., JOHNSON, N., *et al* (1989) Black people and psychiatry in the UK. *Psychiatric Bulletin*, **13**, 482–485
McCLEAN, C. (1994) Accountability. New directions for working in partnership. *Dulwich Centre Newsletters*, **2/3**, 2–5.
NHS MENTAL HEALTH TASK FORCE (1994) *Time for Action Now.* Leeds: NHS Executive.
SMAJE, C. (1995) *Health, Race and Ethnicity – Making Sense of the Evidence.* London: Kings Fund Institute.

21 Alternatives to institutional psychiatry

S. P. SASHIDHARAN

Psychiatric hospitals are dangerous places for psychiatric patients. It has been argued that hospital admissions and hospital-based treatment are not always associated with positive or beneficial outcomes for psychiatric patients and, very often, entry into institutional care works against the interests of service users. There is considerable evidence to support this view, in medical literature and on the basis of the experience of service users (Barton, 1959; Rose, 1986; Rogers *et al*, 1993). Over the past 20 years or so, such a critique of institutional psychiatry has achieved greater popularity than ever before and today very few people doubt the legitimacy of the argument that our psychiatric institutions fall short of the earlier romantic notions that they provide a haven for the vulnerable or cure and care for those in need. Increasingly, psychiatric hospitals, along with their satellite agencies, are identified as coercive institutions mediating a form of social control for the most dispossessed in our society. This can be understood as part of a generalised and more pervasive disciplinary system, primarily concerned with correction and custody (Miller, 1986; Basaglia, 1987; Rogers *et al*, 1993). This view is increasingly reinforced within contemporary discourses around psychiatry, not least from within the oppositional strategies (that is, struggles against institutional psychiatry) and larger political movements involving psychiatric patients or service users (Rose, 1989).

Institutional psychiatry and Black patients

The experience of Black people within European psychiatry has highlighted many problems. For example, the overlap between curative strategies of psychiatry and the custodial functions of psychiatric institutions is most apparent when we consider what happens to minority ethnic groups when they come into contact with European psychiatry. There is a robust body of knowledge that attests to the iniquitous nature of psychiatric interventions in relation to Black people and the coercive nature of psychiatric practice as experienced by minority ethnic groups within Western Europe, particularly in the UK (Cochrane & Sashidharan, 1996; see also Chapters 4, 6 and 7). Although there is a continuing debate about the nature of the problems in this area, there is general agreement that people of non-European origin are over-represented within psychiatric institutions in the UK and that a strong association exists between ethnicity and coercive psychiatric treatment. Furthermore, the diagnostic bias against Black communities, with extreme forms of severe mental illness more likely to be identified within minority ethnic groups, along with the attribution of a greater degree of dangerousness or social pathology in comparison with White groups, is a central theme in this debate. There can be little doubt that the experience of psychiatry by Black patients is substantially different from that of the majority of White patients, with themes of dominance, coercion and control made more explicit and pervasive within most medical practices and clinical procedures, such as diagnosis, hospital admission and treatment.

A clear understanding of how Black people experience psychiatry is impossible without reference to the complex relationship between race and mental disorder within the European imagination. It is not just the common genealogy of the two ideas or the continuous reworking of the two themes to reflect and reinforce each other that allow the approximation and overlap of mental disorder and race, but also the similarity of historical practices brought to bear upon the 'mentally disordered' and the non-European 'races' through the techniques of psychiatry and colonial rule. The most pervasive ideas which ensured the subjugation and the control of people with mental disorders were their segregation from those untainted by mental disorder and the invalidation of mental disorder itself, depriving it of any meaning outside of the medical categories into which 'mental illness' was forced. As with the 'mental science' that provided such legitimacy and power to control 'madness', the 'race science' of the 18th and 19th centuries similarly proved useful in the segregation of non-European from the European people. This was achieved firstly in the colonial context, by the clear boundaries that were drawn across the colonial landscape, separating the coloniser from the colonised and, in parallel, within the imagination and subjectivities of the European, establishing the differences and separateness of Black people, subsequently confirmed as biologically, culturally and socially inferior (Kohn, 1995).

Along with institutionalisation, the emerging science of psychiatry in Europe conferred a new meaning to the experiences of 'madness' and 'deviance' and legitimised the practices of the old asylums, as both beneficial and necessary. Within a post-colonial discourse, the significance of institutions such as mental hospitals, as a repository for the largely unwelcome and mostly unwanted non-Europeans, is easy to understand. Themes of control and coercion, subtly concealed within modern-day psychiatric practices, connect with the experience of Black people living in Europe. The evidence from within psychiatry, the over-representation of Black people within psychiatric hospitals, confirms this, and any analysis of this problem must recognise the ideological links between the treatment of the mentally disordered and the experience of those occupying a similar social and cultural position, namely Black people. In exploring strategic possibilities of change for Black psychiatric patients, the importance of working against psychiatry, or seeking alternatives to the quintessential psychiatric institution such as the hospital, is difficult to ignore.

Alternatives to institutional psychiatry

There already exists a rich seam of theoretical work, analyses and oppositional strategies in relation to alternatives to 'total institutions' such as mental hospitals (Goffman, 1961; Foucault, 1971; Guttari, 1984; Coleman & McLaughlin, 1994). The increasingly sophisticated analysis that confirms the political nature of institutional psychiatry and identifies psychiatric practice, embodied in the role and functions of the mental hospital as a site of struggle for disadvantaged people in general, and Black people in particular, provides the backdrop to professional and popular campaigns to change the nature of psychiatry. The theoretical critique provided by the cultural movement of anti-psychiatry was a significant development in this context but, in the ensuing years, particularly in the past 25 years, the arguments marshalled by Goffman, Laing, Szasz and others became somewhat muted if not totally discredited (Sedgwick, 1982). More recently, however, some of these themes, particularly those which identified the negative and coercive features of psychiatric hospitals, have found renewed expression within the more pragmatic attempts to alter the nature of psychiatric practice. The work of Franco Basgalia and the Democratic Psychiatry movement in Italy is an example of how the ideology of anti-psychiatry was used to bring about fundamental changes within a traditional psychiatric system through a combination of political and professional action (Rotelli, 1988). The main focus of the Italian experience was in seeking and sustaining alternatives to the psychiatric hospital. These reforms, more than anything else, confirmed that it was possible to bring about radical reforms within psychiatry and that professional practice did not necessarily depend on hospitals or asylums.

In the past 25 years, since the start of the Italian reforms, there have been a number of attempts to replicate and further develop such a model, based on a desire to create alternatives to institutional care in a variety of settings (Warner, 1995). In his review, Warner confirms the appropriateness and viability of such initiatives, although most of these have been on a smaller scale than that achieved in Italy. Increasingly, alternative models are informed by the views and aspirations of service users and not merely driven by the ideology of anti-psychiatry (Carling, 1995). Similarly, the professional context in which these changes are brought about requires emphasis and, as Mosher argues, it is no longer a question of whether alternatives to mental hospitals are possible or effective but why we continue to rely on hospital-based models within psychiatry (Mosher, 1983).

The most significant contribution to such an oppositional discourse about psychiatry came initially from Franz Fanon, the French–Caribbean psychiatrist, who was working in Algeria at the time (Fanon, 1965). Fanon's work is critical to any understanding of the relationship between psychiatry and political domination of the colonised by the European coloniser. Although much of his later writing was specifically concerned with emancipatory political action through anti-colonial struggles, Fanon was able to identify a crucial link between psychological illness, being a psychiatric patient and the subjectivities of the colonised. The strain of oppositional thinking that emerged from such an analysis found professional expression in his subsequent work around 'social therapy' which implicitly rejected the need for the custodial institution (Fanon & Azoulay, 1954).

Since Fanon, there have been several attempts to develop further a politically informed psychology around the experience of Black people, particularly based in the post-colonial European context. Although most of this race/psychology discourse remains trapped within predetermined professional boundaries, thus rendering them meaningful only within European paradigms, an increasing dissonance is identified between European cultural and cognitive

forms and the non-European experience (Sashidharan, 1986).
Increasingly, institutional psychiatry is finding it impossible to deal
with both the practical consequences of such clinical practices and
the theoretical and political challenge posed by the intimate
association between psychiatric coercion and ethnicity.

Changing psychiatry

The important question for Black people caught up within psychiatry,
either as patients or as professionals, is how we challenge and change
the current situation. If we do not accept that psychiatry is a politically
neutral activity or, for that matter, a benign discipline, on a par
with other health care activities, then the only meaningful position
that we can adopt is one that is opposed to the interests of psychiatry.
However, a theoretical analysis along these lines by itself does
not alter the experience of Black people within psychiatry. The
continuing marginalisation of Black people within psychiatry and
the invalidation of Black people's life experiences through a
combination of medical technologies and powerful social sanctions,
both incorporated into the apparently seamless strategies of mental
health care, require a challenge that goes beyond the rhetoric of
largely discredited anti-psychiatry. As the experience of Black
voluntary initiatives within mental health care shows, alternative
practices and practical remedies to the current crisis must be
explored (Francis *et al*, 1989; Kareem & Littlewood, 1989).

The move towards alternatives to psychiatric hospitals provides a
unique opportunity to reappraise the validity of current models of
care as well as establishing viable alternatives even within circum-
scribed areas of professional activity. The financial and professional
constraints that made any change impossible until quite recently
have been loosened and as psychiatric practice is brought under
increasing scrutiny, both within the public and professional arena,
the arguments for alternative practice have become irresistible. The
failure of psychiatry, at least for Black people, is clearly visible and
the impatience to change the practices and procedures of psychiatry
is no longer confined to a small group of activists or the Black
community.

The Ladywood experience

Ladywood is a typical electoral ward in an inner city area in
Birmingham. Like many other urban settings in England, Ladywood

is characterised by high levels of social and material deprivation, according to all the indices of urban deprivation. Long-term unemployment, poor quality housing, multiple-occupancy dwellings impoverished educational and social facilities are some of the more obvious examples of this. In addition, the local communities in such inner city settings are becoming increasingly alienated and fragmented, with little in the way of real opportunities for education or work. It is typical of such inner city areas in this country that a significant proportion of the local population is from Black and minority ethnic backgrounds. Ladywood is no exception to this, and nearly half of the local residents are Black or Asian in origin.

The general rule that the levels of mental distress in a given population are significantly correlated with indices of social deprivation also applies to Ladywood. Such an association holds true for all forms of mental disorder, including the most severe manifestations, such as psychotic illnesses. Figures for Ladywood confirm this. For example, a recent survey of the local services revealed that the prevalence of serious mental illness was known to local psychiatric services in the electoral wards of Ladywood and South Soho to be 6–10 times higher than those reported elsewhere (Northern Birmingham Mental Health Trust, 1996). The observation that nearly 2 in 100 of the local population are in touch with local services for the treatment of a severe mental illness confirms the extent to which the local community is already involved in psychiatric services – but this also underlines the severe nature of the mental health problems experienced by psychiatric patients locally.

Like many other inner city areas in this country, mental health care for the local population in Ladywood is provided through a traditional mental hospital. This hospital, built as the local lunatic asylum in 1848, is typical of the large Victorian institutions which continue to dominate psychiatric care in most urban settings in this country. Situated adjacent to the local prison, All Saints Hospital gradually became a significant landmark locally, dominating the lives of increasingly large numbers of the population of Ladywood and the surrounding areas. After the heyday of asylum-based care in psychiatry (at one time the hospital housed more than 1000 patients), All Saints Hospital, like many other hospitals, underwent major changes, such as a gradual reduction in the number of beds and a restriction of 'therapeutic' activities. These changes were heavily influenced by the emergence of a more explicitly medical approach in the treatment of mental disorders, with the advent of newer psychotropic drugs and the rapid growth of a more 'scientific' psychiatry. It was also at around this time that the local people became aware that a disproportionate number of Black people were being admitted to the hospital. The pattern of psychiatric care in Ladywood remained largely the same over the next three decades. By the late 1980s, mental health care in Ladywood had become further restricted and almost exclusively confined to the local psychiatric hospital. For example, over 90% of the resources available were confined to one acute admission ward within this hospital, providing in-patient care for a total of 22 patients at any one time. There was very little in the way of mental health care available outside of the confines of the hospital and the institution had become increasingly remote from the local community. Within the imagination of the local people, the in-patient unit dealing with Ladywood patients and the local hospital were identified as strange and forbidding places which relatives or friends got 'put into' if their behaviour caused problems outside in the community.

In communities such as Ladywood a different dimension has been added to the already fraught relationship between the local people and psychiatric institutions. This is the demographic shift, following the arrival of immigrants from Ireland, followed by Asian and Caribbean people, who settled in the deprived urban areas. Economic and social factors have always played a major part in the settlement of immigrant communities in these neighbourhoods and localities. Such factors have continued to exert a powerful influence in sustaining a segregated pattern of ethnic settlement in places like Birmingham, and over the years the inner city, with its mental hospital and the prison, has become almost synonymous with Black presence in England. However, it is not just this geographical proximity that brought about an intimacy between the local Black population and psychiatric institutions. In the wake of the post-war migration of Caribbean and Asian people to the UK, most urban psychiatric hospitals began to reflect the demographic shifts in the local population, with a significant Black presence in hospital admissions. Furthermore, local communities began to voice their concern about the disproportionate numbers of Black people who were deemed as requiring the attention of such institutional agencies. For example, when the first voluntary mental health initiative by the Black community was set up in Brixton in the late 1970s (the African–Caribbean Mental Health Association), one of the observations made by the group of women who organised themselves in this way was that most families in the local community had at least one of their members 'locked up' in the local psychiatric hospital. Subsequent academic research, and the politicisation of Black mental health which followed, quickly confirmed that psychiatry, like policing, was becoming an area of struggle for Black people in the UK (Mercer, 1986).

The ensuing debate and arguments about the nature of psychiatric practice as it impinged on minority groups increasingly identified mental hospitals at the centre of such concerns. Medical or psychiatric discourse and the more general but highly politicised analysis about the racialisation of psychiatric theory and practice both shared this view (Black Health Workers and Patients Group, 1983; Miller, 1986). Partly, this arose out of the immediacy and greater visibility of hospital-based psychiatric practice, in terms of coercive admissions, forcible treatment and the marginalisation of Black patients' needs. However, the focus on psychiatric hospitals was also influenced by the fact that the experience of psychiatry by Black people, until the advent of community care, was predominantly confined to institutional settings. The question that was being asked, both within psychiatric research and by the Black communities, through the various self-help and other voluntary initiatives, was why Black people were over-represented in psychiatric hospitals and why hospital-based practice appeared to discriminate and disadvantage Black patients. The negative impact and sometimes tragic consequences of psychiatric treatment were also seen fundamentally as a product of institutional treatment, usually of a compulsory nature. For example, it is highly relevant that, until quite recently, psychiatric research in relation to Black people's mental health in the UK has been conducted exclusively around psychiatric hospitals (Cochrane & Sashidharan, 1996).

It was in this political and intellectual climate that the events leading to the closure of acute in-patient facilities in Ladywood and the creation of alternative practices such as 'home treatment' must be understood. By the late 1980s, institutional treatment for mental disorders had become almost untenable and, in practice, unsustainable in the inner city, given the hostility to the mental hospital and the rejection of hospital care by the local Black community and Black service users. Similarly, the tensions and pressures created within the hospital environment by the active resistance to any form of therapy by Black patients and the consequent sense of opposition and confrontation that imbued every transaction between patients and staff made the idea of treatment or care almost meaningless. There was, of course, the view that the problems of over-representation of Black people within psychiatric facilities and the excess diagnosis of serious mental illness and coercive treatment were primarily related to a real excess of mental illness among communities of African origin and that the solutions to these could be found in clinical and public health strategies, well tested and well established in other areas. Such an analysis was, of course, necessary and helpful within a medical discourse which suggested that mental illness and its treatment were somehow located outside of the social and political context within which mental disorder was being created and subjugated through psychiatry. According to this view, psychiatric practice is essentially a medical matter transacted through the technologies of medicine. Therefore, the political and intellectual tensions that are made visible within an inner city practice are, at worst, tangential to the real business of treating mental illnesses or, at best, a product of a kind of cultural dissonance arising out of the inability of non-European people to accept the prevailing ideologies around care and treatment.

Home treatment – the process of change

Given the iniquitous nature of psychiatric care in Ladywood and the general recognition that the problems with clinical practice could be traced to the nature of acute hospital care in that setting, it was not difficult to recognise the need for alternative strategies to deal with admissions to the hospital. However, the professional acceptance of such a view was fraught with difficulty. To a large extent, professional training and practice in the area of mental health are a product of our institutional history, and our theories and perspectives are derived from observing and containing mental disorder in an institutional setting. Because of that, any invitation to reappraise, if not abandon, the need for psychiatric hospitals as the central location of our practice carried with it an implicit assumption that we would have to change the way we deal with mental disorder in our respective professional roles. Such a threat to our historically determined positions in the business of caring for the mentally ill was further augmented by the relative lack of understanding, both in theoretical and practical terms, about how we would continue to work as mental health professionals. The anxieties expressed by the staff, therefore, needed to be resolved before we could bring about the closure of the hospital ward. This was achieved, at least to some extent, by regular staff group meetings which provided the opportunity to voice concerns and renew our commitment to developing alternative practices.

This process would have been incomplete, if not impossible to achieve, without the active collaboration and support of local community groups, psychiatric service users and their relatives, and the voluntary mental health groups, especially those from within the Black community. It is often the case that the mental health initiatives from outside the governmental sector or the statutory agencies, especially if they are led by service users, occupy a position opposed to that of traditional psychiatry and related agencies. In many ways, the strength of such organisations lies in their ability to challenge and confront professional agencies, and in tilting the balance of power within orthodox psychiatry in favour of service users and away from institutions such as mental hospitals. One of the most significant developments in the area of mental health service provision, especially around the issue of race and ethnicity, has been the emergence of politically informed Black voluntary agencies, both as service providers and as single-issue pressure groups (see Chapter 20). Many people working inside traditional psychiatry, mostly as professionals, had identified the need to become involved with such community groups, working on the outside, as a way of bringing about the possibility of change, especially for Black people (Black Health Workers and Patients Group, 1983). For example, groups such as the National Ethnic Minority Health Care Group, the Black Patients and Workers Group based in London and the Harambee Organisation in Birmingham, set up in the 1970s, had all become involved in seeking practical solutions to the problems that Black people were experiencing within psychiatry. As these organisations became invested with increasing community support, they provided an opportunity for many Black professionals to become involved in their work, thus enabling many such people to work both from the inside and the outside at the same time. Suddenly there was a channel from the community into the hospital, often breaching the traditional boundaries within which a segregated psychiatry operated.

In Ladywood, the move towards ward closure was facilitated by the persistent and often impatient demand for change from the local Black community. Local groups such as Harambee, an organisation originally set up to deal with the problems of homelessness among young African–Caribbeans, and Handsworth Community Care Group, another Black voluntary initiative that provided support for Black service users through a day-care facility in the basement of a local church, had long argued that mental health services should address the specific needs of Black and other ethnic minority groups. Initially the demand for appropriate and adequate services for Black people had been focused on hospital care and the negative nature of much of the hospital care.

Mental health professionals including psychiatrists, nurses and social workers were increasingly disenchanted with their inability to transform existing services, partly as a result of the new management ethos within the health service, and it was critical to recognise the opportunity that existed to build political alliances with community groups at large. In Ladywood, the militancy and commitment shown by the local groups not only facilitated plans to move away from traditional structures of service provision, but also ensured that the new services would have the full support of the community. One key development in making the new service acceptable to the local community was setting up joint meetings with the organisations involved with mental health as well as involving other agencies, such as Black churches, gurdwaras and the local mosque, in the ongoing debate about what the local community wanted and what those working in the health service could provide. Once these alliances were built and nurtured, it was only a question of time before the hospital base was abandoned.

The final hurdle that remained, apart from the question of professional leadership, concerned the new form of mental health practice that would replace the old institutional model. It is often easier to identify the problems and limitations of institutional practice, especially when the contradiction at the heart of psychiatric practice between custody and care or cure and control is made explicit, than to seek appropriate solutions to those problems. The service users in Ladywood and most of their relatives or carers had identified a 24-hour service, aimed at dealing with crisis situations, as the priority. They had also expressed a clear preference for such a service to be available in the community rather than in the hospital. This model, of course, had been well tested in a variety of settings and the benefits of such interventions amply illustrated in existing psychiatric literature. However, shifting the acute services entirely into the community and providing all aspects of acute care in people's homes presented a fundamental dilemma.

The most persuasive argument was that clinical practice, including what psychiatric doctors and nurses normally did in the hospital setting, could be carried out, often more effectively, without the need for compulsion and hospital admission. According to this analysis, the only thing that the hospital offered, over and above what could be achieved in the normal living environment of psychiatric patients, was the element of control and coercion that is invested in professional practice.

Once again, such an understanding would not have been easily available to us if we were operating outside of the racial and ethnic context provided by inner city psychiatry. What came out of it was a confidence that we would be able to locate our practice outside of a coercive framework within which the need for acute care was often equated with the need for hospital admission. The physical removal of the patients that this entailed, from their normal living environment into a hospital, was often resisted – but such resistance was invariably understood by psychiatry as further evidence of mental disorder and the need for removal. In the highly racialised and confrontational environment within which psychiatry operated in inner city Birmingham, clinical practice had become secondary to, if not part of, social control, both within the imagination of the local community and in the perceptions of Black service users. The only way to break this cycle of suspicion, mutual distrust, professional prejudice and, to some extent, inertia on the part of service providers was to deny psychiatrists the basis of professional power, the coercive strategies and compulsory powers invested in hospital admission.

Impact of home treatment on psychiatric services

The acute in-patient ward serving the catchment area of Ladywood and South Soho was closed down on 14 July 1990 and home treatment was initiated as an alternative form of acute care. The principles underpinning the new service are summarised in Box 1.

Home treatment has been available in this locality over the past eight years and has become the central feature of acute services locally. For a period of four years, between 1992 and 1995, the service was expanded to cover the whole of the health district (population of under 200 000), but the number of places available on home treatment was restricted to a maximum of 15 during this time, mainly because of limited resources. Since 1996, however, the service has

---

Box 1
Principles of home treatment

Avoid hospitalisation – abandon the reliance on hospital beds
Provide a 24-hour service
Carry out assessment and treatment at home
Engage with users and carers
Apply non-coercive interventions
Apply needs-based assessment instead of medical diagnosis
Care plans should be shared with users and carers
Employ multi-disciplinary working
Work jointly with community agencies including voluntary groups, churches,
    mosques and temples
Use non-medical models of explanation and theory

become re-focused on Ladywood, where it is once again acting as a screen for all potential admissions to hospital.

The data presented here refer to the first two years of the service, between July 1990 and June 1992, when the main objective of the service was to prevent hospital admissions to Ladywood. The impact of a new service should not be measured in terms of changes in the nature of service activity (such as hospital admission rate) but, more significantly, whether community-based interventions have an influence on clinical practice and professional outlook in general. As I have already argued, unless we change the way we conceptualise psychological distress and understand it fully in contextual terms, our ability to alter the current iniquitous pattern of service delivery, especially in relation to disadvantaged groups, will remain seriously compromised.

Impact on service delivery

Data can be presented in relation to three areas of service activity, all related to acute care and the management of severe mental illness and other crisis conditions that usually require hospital admission: first, the impact of home treatment on local hospital admission rates; second, the degree to which the new service was targeted to those with severe mental illness; and third, the extent to which the new service treated people successfully at home, that is, the proportion of people with acute psychiatric problems who had to be admitted to the psychiatric hospital because they could not be managed successfully at home. All three questions are significant in the context of providing an alternative to hospital admission to Black people.

Hospital admission rates

There was an immediate and significant reduction in hospital admissions from the catchment area as soon as the alternative service was set up. The average number of admissions to hospital for the age group 18–65 years declined by 50% once home treatment became available and this trend was maintained subsequently (see Fig. 1). Although the number of admissions to in-patient care decreased after an alternative to hospital admission became available, Fig. 1 also shows that during this period the demand for acute care was not reduced. The admissions shown here include those admitted from within the home treatment programme as well as a smaller

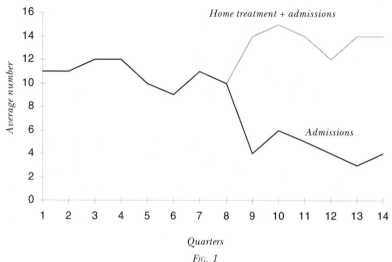

Fig. 1
Quarterly averages of hospital admissions and home treatment combined with hospital admissions

number of individuals who gained direct entry into in-patient care, bypassing the home treatment service.

Targeting of home treatment

One of the anxieties concerning psychiatric emergency services specifically targeted at reducing in-patient bed usage is that such services may become focused on those who are not currently seen as high users of in-patient services, namely those with diagnostic conditions other than severe mental illness. This should be an important consideration in the context of setting up community services in general. For example, a recent audit of community mental health teams (CMHTs) in England showed that the case load of CMHTs had considerable variations, particularly the proportion of patients with severe and enduring mental health problems.

Table 1 shows the diagnostic distribution of all those included in the home treatment sample over the first two years. This confirms that nearly three-quarters of the episodes of acute care undertaken by home treatment were for conditions such as schizophrenia, paranoid psychosis and major depression and less than 20% were for those with no identifiable severe mental illness, experiencing

TABLE 1
Diagnosis distribution in the home treatment group

Main diagnosis (ICD–10)	*n* (216)	%
Organic mental disorder (F00–09)	7	3.2
Psychoactive substance abuse, including alcohol (F10–19)	11	5.1
Schizophrenia and delusional disorders (F20–29)	77	35.7
Manic episode (F30)	49	22.7
Depressive episode (F32–39)	24	11.1
Neurotic, stress-related and somatoform disorders (F40–48)	48	22.2

psychosocial crisis. The successful targeting of home treatment to those with severe mental illness was achieved as a result of setting up the service as a filter for all potential hospital admissions from the area and not as an adjunct to an existing in-patient service. In the latter case, it is likely that the channel leading to hospital admission will remain largely unsupervised and the new service will therefore meet the needs of users who are not necessarily making demands on current in-patient services.

Outcome of home treatment

Table 2 shows the outcome of home treatment in the 216 episodes of acute care. The two important findings are that, first, less than 20% of the episodes resulted in hospital admission as part of their acute care and, second, that the majority of users remain in contact with services at the end of their acute care. The chances of hospital admission were greatest for those with a diagnosis of manic illness and least for those without severe mental illness. However, when risk of hospital admission is examined in those with a diagnosis of psychosis or severe mental illness, the proportion that resulted in hospital admission was still under 20%, showing that four out of

TABLE 2
Outcome of home treatment

Outcome	*n*	%
Hospital admission (voluntary)	14	6.5
Hospital admission (under the Mental Health Act)	19	8.8
Time-limited out-patient follow-up	51	23.6
Longer term psychiatric follow-up	116	53.7
Referral to specialist services	10	4.6
No psychiatric follow-up	6	2.8

five people with severe mental illness, who may end up in hospital during the acute phase of their episode, can be successfully treated at home if an alternative, community-based service is made available.

Conclusions

Although the experience of Black people within psychiatry and the racially discriminatory nature of mental health care systems in general continue to dominate the discourse around psychiatry and race in this country, there have been very few practical solutions to the problems identified within clinical practice.

On the whole, attempts to make psychiatric practice more sensitive to the needs of Black people appear to have had little impact on clinical practice in general. For example, it would be very difficult to argue that the experience of psychiatry by Black people has changed very much in the past three decades or so, despite the salience given to cultural and ethnic issues through the resuscitation of transcultural psychiatry as an academic discipline, the managerial commitment to make services ethnically sensitive and the demands for a radical reappraisal of psychiatric care from anti-racist perspectives. The disciplinary and regulatory functions of psychiatry, as embodied in institutional practices, have hardly changed as a result of such reforms or resistant ideologies. Unless the institutional model which underpins much of psychiatric practice in this country is effectively challenged, the segregation and invalidation of those deemed deviant, in cultural, social and medical terms, will continue. As we have already seen, the people who are adversely affected by the regulatory and disciplining practices, transacted through the medical technologies of psychiatry, are more likely to be those deemed marginal or otherwise excluded from the centre.

By acknowledging the fundamental importance of the psychiatric hospital or the asylum in mediating psychiatric practice, particularly the more correctional and punitive aspects of clinical practice, we were identifying the need to work against the hospital as well as seeking alternative practices. At a very local level we were able to initiate a professional move in this direction, bringing about some fundamental changes in the way psychiatry operated in that particular environment. More than the creation of an alternative service, in the way of home treatment, what this has achieved is the possibility that psychiatric services in our inner city areas could begin to address issues around care and cure rather than continue to be biased in favour of custody and control.

References

BARTON, W. R. (1959) *Institutional Neurosis*. Bristol: John Wright & Sons.

BASAGLIA, F. (1987) *Psychiatry Inside Out: Selected Writings of Franco Basaglia*. New York: Columbia University Press.

BLACK HEALTH WORKERS AND PATIENTS GROUP (1983) Psychiatry and the corporate stake. *Race and Class*, **25**, 49–64.

CARLING, P. J. (1995) *Return to Community. Building Support Systems for People with Psychiatric Disabilities*. New York: Guilford.

COCHRANE, R. & SASHIDHARAN, S. P. (1996) Mental health and ethnic minorities: a review of the literature and implications for services. In *Ethnicity and Health*, CRD Report 5. York: NHS Centre for Reviews and Dissemination. Social Policy Research Unit, University of York.

COLEMAN, R. & MCLAUGHLIN, T. (1994) I'm back! In support of resisting treatment. *Asylum*, **8**, 26–28.

FANON, F. (1965) *The Wretched of the Earth* (trans. C. Farrington). New York: Grove Press.

—— & AZOULAY, J. (1954) *La Socialtheraphie dans un Service d'Hommes Musulmans, Difficulties Methodologiques*, L'Information Psychiatrique 4me serie. 9. Paris: Hôpital Psychiatrique de Blida-Joinvillé.

FOUCAULT, M. (1971) *Madness and Civilisation*. London: Tavistock.

FRANCIS, E., DAVID, J., JOHNSON, N., *et al* (1989) Black people and psychiatry in the UK. An alternative to institutional care. *Psychiatric Bulletin*, **13**, 482–485.

GOFFMAN, E. (1961) *Asylums: Essays on the Social Situation of Mental Patients*. New York: Doubleday.

GUTTARI, F. (1984) *Molecular Revolution: Psychiatry and Politics*. Harmondsworth: Peregrine.

KAREEM, J. & LITTLEWOOD, R. (1989) *Intercultural Therapy: Theory and Practice*. Oxford: Blackwell.

KOHN, M. (1995) *The Race Gallery. The Return of Racial Science*. London: Jonathan Cape.

MERCER, K. (1986) Racism and transcultural psychiatry. In *The Power of Psychiatry* (eds P. Miller & N. Rose), pp. 112–142. Cambridge: Polity Press.

MILLER, P. (1986) Critiques of psychiatry and critical sociologies of madness. In *The Power of Psychiatry*, pp. 12–42. Cambridge: Polity Press.

MOODLEY, P. (1993) Setting up services for ethnic minorities. In *Principles of Social Psychiatry*. (eds D. Bhugra & J. Leff), pp. 490–501. Oxford: Blackwell.

MOSHER, L. R. (1983) Alternatives to psychiatric hospitalisation: why has research failed to be translated into practice? *New England Journal of Medicine*, **309**, 1579–1580.

NORTHERN BIRMINGHAM MENTAL HEALTH TRUST (1996) *Results of the 'Stock-Take' of People in Touch with Local Psychiatry Service*. Birmingham: Northern Birmingham Mental Health Trust.

PARKER, I., GEORGACA, E., HARPER, D., *et al* (1995) *Deconstructing Psychopathology*. London: Sage.

ROGERS, A., PILGRIM, D. & LACEY, R. (1993) *Experiencing Psychiatry. Users' Views of Psychiatry*. London: MIND.

ROSE, N. (1986) Psychiatry: the discipline of mental health. In *The Power of Psychiatry* (eds P. Miller & N. Rose), pp. 43–84. Cambridge: Polity Press.

—— (1989) *Governing the Soul: Technologies of Human Subjectivity*. London: Routledge.

ROTELLI, F. (1988) Changing psychiatric services in Italy. In *Psychiatry in Transition. The British and Italian Experiences* (ed. S. Ramon), pp. 182–190. London: Pluto Press.

SASHIDHARAN, S. P. (1986) The ideology and politics of transcultural psychiatry. In *Transcultural Psychiatry* (ed. J. Cox), pp. 158–178. London: Croom Helm.

SEDGWICK, P. (1982) *Psychopolitics*. London: Pluto Press.

WARNER, R. (ed.) (1995) *Alternatives to the Hospital for Acute Psychiatric Treatment*. Washington, DC: American Psychiatric Association.

22 Service provision for ethnic minorities

KAMALDEEP BHUI and DINESH BHUGRA

Ethnic minorities in the UK experience discrimination and specific physical and mental ill health problems, yet they do not have equal access to health and social services (see Chapters 2 and 21). The core mental health needs of ethnic minorities are similar to those reported by the White majority, but among ethnic minorities there are additional factors which significantly influence the presentation, assessment and management process. Our aim here is to focus attention on the structural and operational characteristics of services, which for different ethnic minority groups fashion patterns of service utilisation and accessibility.

Terminology

We use the term 'ethnic minorities' to represent all racial and cultural minorities in order to clarify those service provision issues common to groups as diverse as the Chinese, Asian or African–Caribbean communities (also see Chapter 1). Common inferences which we wish to avoid are: (a) the use of the term ethnic minorities to create the illusion that all ethnic minorities are homogenous and that the solution to the problems of access to health and social care are singular for all groups; (b) that all ethnic minority groups have such similar historical experiences and that their experience of adversity or affluence are not dissimilar across generational, geographical, racial and cultural boundaries; and (c) that ethnic minorities have similar expectations and needs from health services. Sashidharan (1993) argues cogently that the application of Odegaard's model of migratory stresses to the ethnic minorities is not to be recommended. The historical reasons for migration for any one cultural group may affect only a small proportion of ethnic minority individuals in the UK. For example, the needs of refugees are different and their political reasons for migration create a unique set of circumstances which influence types of psychiatric disorder and provision of the necessary interventions.

Rates of disorder and the schizophrenia debate

The diagnostic conundrum of psychiatric illnesses in ethnic minorities remains a very important issue. Several studies in the UK have shown high rates of schizophrenia in African–Caribbean people (see Chapter 5) although the ethnocentric diagnosis of such a condition along with methodological problems in data collection, as well as generalisation from a small number of cases, have produced a deserved degree of concern from the African–Caribbean community (see Chapters 5 and 6). Adebimpe (1994) has demonstrated that data from the Epidemiological Catchment Area Study, after correction for age, gender, socio-economic status and marital status, demonstrate that there is no significant difference in rates of schizophrenia. Gillam *et al* (1989) have argued that ethnic minorities in the UK are less likely to receive diagnoses of anxiety or depression in primary care (see Chapter 7). It can be hypothesised that these communities would be expected to have higher rates of these conditions, which are closely linked with stress-related disorders as well as major psychotic illnesses. Thus, two problems begin to emerge. First, the acceptance that the rate of schizophrenia is truly higher among the African–Caribbean community in the UK, even though this has been shown not to be a consistent finding in other ethnic minority groups; and second, whether low rates of presentation of anxiety and depression are genuinely low, or whether these findings reflect inequitable access to and utilisation of services. There may, of course, be a possibility that members of ethnic minorities deal with their anxiety and depression using complementary or alternative means (Nazroo, 1997; see Chapter 23). Therefore, it is vital to ascertain their explanatory models to determine their current and potential use of services. Although initial steps have been taken in this direction (Lloyd, 1993; also Chapter 7) more needs to be done in determining incidence, prevalence, methods of help-seeking and explanatory models of distress states and psychiatric disorders.

Service provision

The basic principle of providing community services (especially if they are state-provided) is that of equitable provision to all users

---

Box 1
Local information directories

(a)   Providers should disseminate information on local services covering: legal rights, medication, meanings of diagnoses, treatment packages, advocacy, support agencies, social services, resource centres and facilities available.

(b)   Black mental health organisations should provide information about the services available, crisis centres, languages spoken, matching local population profiles, links with social and statutory organisations.

(c)   Religious and cultural groups.

(d)   Interpreting agencies should be available and should: be gender/culture-specific; have a policy of ease of availability; have guidelines and training for their staff; be confidential.

(Bhugra, 1993*b*). There must be a way of ascertaining specific areas of need in order to provide a service which can deliver the intervention which best meets that need (see Chapter 15). Measures taken will not succeed if the necessary range of service structural components of a comprehensive mental health service are absent.

For any kind of service provision, especially in the community, public health education campaigns form an important part. The delivery of such education needs to be carried out in innovative and local ways. Information on local services must include factors like local agencies and primary and secondary services (see Box 1).

Multi-professional forums for eliciting opinions from the community as well as local users should form the backbone of the services. A directory of local mental health agencies should be readily available in GP surgeries, local libraries and other public places, as well as through schools, hospitals and other organisations.

Treatment preferences by people from ethnic minority groups must be given consideration along with an assessment of risk related to a particular decision informing the eventual outcome. Individual choice of treatment should be respected if at all possible, irrespective of the ethnic origin of the user (see Box 2).

Good practice must include taking into account cultural and religious preferences of patients and regular family meetings throughout patient contact, especially if the patient's needs dictate such contact. Mental illness may affect or prevent individuals from fulfilling their social role, and the individual's distress may be experienced as family distress. Such a social role must be supported to the advantage of the patient and the family. Purchasers may wish to look at this in conjunction with

---

Box 2
Multi-professional forums – arrangements to be made when meeting with ethnic groups

How often should the meetings be held?
Who should attend the meetings?
Who should set the agenda and decide whether a chairperson is required?
Ensure that local agencies are represented.
Ensure that the community is represented – be aware which specific groups
   are represented.
Local views should be taken into account. Establish how this can be done. If it
   is not possible, find out why not.
Are specific guidelines being dealt with?
Actively implement policies.
Establish whether any specialist agencies are involved.
Assess which groups are not accounted for.

---

other psychotherapies (see Box 3). However, there may be key
differences between the second generation and the older population (Bhugra & Bhui, 1998a).

Principles

All services need to be local, accessible, comprehensive, flexible and
consumer-orientated, empowering those using the services. They
must be focused on their strengths and be accountable and racially
and culturally appropriate (Strathdee & Thornicroft, 1993).
Strathdee & Thornicroft (1993) advocate the National Institute of
Mental Health plan which involves needs-led, component-led
functional models of service development. Such a model can be
applied to ethnic minorities but has to work from the bottom
upwards.

Box 3
Family therapy and psychotherapies

Establish the percentage of patients having family meetings.
Is there a racial and cultural breakdown?
Is the patient involved?
Ascertain whether family meetings are part of treatment packages.
Are there arrangements for intercultural family therapy?
Are there any trained family therapists?
There should be a local evaluation of family therapies.
Discover who is not offered therapy and why not.

With an increasing emphasis on sectorisation, informed decisions and necessary services can only be delivered if there are appropriate epidemiological data defining the population's demographics as well as the prevalence of psychiatric disorders. Procedures to collect data need to be incorporated into the planning processes with a mechanism to ensure that data collection is repeated at regular intervals in order to account for changes in the population (Bhui *et al*, 1995*a*); invariably, areas of deprivation with higher rates of psychiatric disorders and a more mobile population have higher rates of resident ethnic minorities. The basic information systems addressing the size of the local populations, local vulnerabilities, known rates of disorder and indices of deprivation are essential (Bhui *et al*, 1995*a*). Only then will service planners and providers be in a position to approach the planning of future developments.

The greater emphasis on community-based health care has brought its own challenges. Often the plan has been to move service components into the community with little thought being given to how these relocated service components can be of greater use. We outline some of the factors essential for a successful transition into community care.

Primary care interface

One of the priority tasks when planning community-based services is the development between the purchaser, commissioners and other stakeholders of a common vision and statement regarding the role of hospital care, day care, primary care and home-based treatments. The services should be comprehensive, collaborative and cooperative and need to be coterminous with social service boundaries (Bhugra *et al*, 1995). It is crucial to link developing community mental health services into a comprehensive framework including primary care, non-statutory organisations, health care provided by statutory services and social care provided by social services. One of the major features of health care in the UK is the almost universal availability of primary health care. As discussed in Chapters 4 and 19, Goldberg & Huxley (1980) demonstrated that of 1000 people in the population one-quarter experienced symptoms, during a period of a year, which could be classified as psychological or psychiatric. Of these, 230 presented to their general practitioner, 17 were referred to psychiatrists and six were admitted to hospital. Hence, it becomes important to strengthen links with primary care (see Chapters 3 and 4). It has been argued that patients can be divided into three groups: those who require general medical intervention; those seeking non-specialist local psychiatric help;

and those who require specialist psychiatric care (Bennett & Freeman, 1991). A major advantage of liaison with primary care services is their accessibility and proximity and that the consultation itself can be less stigmatising. The links with local general practices can be developed at various levels depending upon the profile of needs that patients present with. The presentation of patients who have common psychiatric disorders like anxiety or depression may be linked to somatisation or comorbid physical disorder. This is true across various ethnic groups and is not a pathognomonic observation in ethnic minorities. A further group of patients includes those with eating disorders, obsessional disorders and episodic psychotic illnesses. The final group comprises people with chronic and usually disabling illnesses also subsumed by the term 'chronic severe mental illness'. Although the general emphasis in some community psychiatric services has been on patients with chronic severe mental illness, the group of patients with neurotic disorders cause much concern to their general practitioners and there are significant costs due to their disability. It may be argued that this particular group is the most likely to be missed with regard to ethnic minorities. However, the literature shows that the rates of neurotic disorder in the community may be lower than expected (Nazroo, 1997).

Primary-care-based specialist services have to deal with emergencies as well as routine referral services. As Strathdee (1994) has outlined, rapid crisis response, contact with specialist services and home-based assessments are the foundations of successful primary care services. The role of community psychiatric nurses and/or psychologists in this context is determined by the number and the needs of the patients. Joint shared care registers for those with chronic severe mental illness encourage a quick response to acute crises.

Specialist mental health services

Specialist services in the community should include: general adult, rehabilitation (continuing care), forensic, liaison, substance misuse, older adult, young child and adolescent services, as well as different kinds of psychotherapy services. The use of case managers and keyworkers is discussed by Strathdee & Thornicroft (1993). Both hospital and community-based services have little control over the numbers and type of patients they encounter, yet they may have to prioritise. Some type of prioritisation may work well if it is operationally defined in partnership with other local service providers. The aims of the local mental health services need to be clearly conceptualised along with the needs of the service users. Standards of care (by the purchasers) should be specified and monitoring of the provision of services (by both purchasers and providers) along with meaningful evaluation of the outcomes should take place(Bennett & Freeman, 1991). As Bennett & Freeman emphasise, a very important aspect of community care is that much of the conventional dyadic relationship between the doctor and patient is replaced by a relationship with the multi-disciplinary professional team. Different members of the team have different skills and levels of expertise and are able to provide an almost complete biopsychosocial model of management. The use of multi-disciplinary team members with ethnic minorities has not been studied, but it would be useful to understand the perceptions of patients and their carers about specific members of the team. Furthermore, the work carried out by multi-disciplinary team members has to be adapted when applying a biopsychosocial model to ethnic minority patients, for whom such a psychiatric model may be alien. Their health may be influenced more by poverty, economic and social disadvantage and discrimination and differing health beliefs. This observation needs to be confirmed in a more rigorous scientific fashion and the training of the members of multi-disciplinary teams will have to alter accordingly. Within the provisions of community care, there remains a mandate for providing a 'safe haven' where a patient, who may have terrible experiences related to his or her psychopathology, can be looked after and cared for.

The community care plan in *Caring for People* (Department of Health, 1989) came into effect on 1 April 1993. This document sets out the blueprint for community care, the basic tenet being that services should be adapted to the needs of the individual rather than the other way around (see Chapter 15). The NHS and Community Care Act 1989 reflected some of the ambivalence of the government in setting up community care services. Although the main objective of the Act is to develop and improve ways of providing community services, it underplays the need for supervised accommodation either in residential care home or nursing home settings. Local authorities are expected to set eight key tasks and are obliged to report on their progress (Bhugra *et al*, 1995). It is likely that minority ethnic groups will benefit from changes proposed in the recent NHS White Papers, which encourage the development of a more primary-care-led service framework. Single-gender wards and availability of alternative or complementary therapies are likely to result from this.

Shaping services to meet the needs of ethnic minorities

There are several issues regarding ethnic minorities' service needs that must be addressed prior to setting up the services that the patients and their carers will use. It is necessary to identify a mechanism for measuring need appropriately and quickly (see Chapter 15). A good starting point is the collation of detailed information on age, gender and generational and cultural structures of the local population. In inner cities especially this may change fairly rapidly. Valid measures of population and individual need must be validated and utilised with the support and participation of local ethnic minority populations. As Bhui *et al* (1995*a*) have cautioned, such an ideological exercise of developing a multicultural needs assessment may fail because specific factors are being ignored – these may include a lack of known effective interventions; unavailability of appropriate interventions; ignorance of cultural factors and needs such as religious norms; language difficulties; and a lack of scientific information on potential treatments that the patients and their carers may wish for. Each cultural group may place unique demands on service provider units, stretching their established (by necessity, in the statutory sector) evidence-based range of interventions. The potential problems are illustrated in Tables 1 and 2. Any service provider needs to think through approaches to adopt with patients who fall into one of the conflict groups as it is these patients for whom existing services do not have a solution.

Alternative treatments are increasingly being requested by people with mental health problems, yet the absence of randomised controlled trials demonstrating efficacy deters statutory services from using such interventions. One might argue that statutory services

TABLE 1
Potential needs assessment outcomes for any single intervention

Professional judgement	Patient	Conflict?
Requires intervention	Demands intervention	No
Does not require intervention	Demands intervention	Yes[1]
Requires intervention	Refuses intervention	Yes[1]
Does not require intervention	Does not demand intervention	No
No effective intervention	Demands treatment	Yes[1]

1. Inherent in any medical evaluation is that all interventions are known about; medical interventions are the most efficacious, and alternative treatments may be used only if there is scientific evidence of its success. Individual patients may find some interventions or coping strategies immensely helpful but these may not be acknowledged by professionals.

TABLE 2
Problems for ethnic minorities after a needs assessment

The intervention being demanded may not be clinically indicated	*Example:* Admission to hospital when a family is in crisis and family therapy work is available (this assumes that an accurate assessment of an individual is possible and that it takes account of differences in culture). The demand must be motivated by the needs of the patient or family and warrants evaluation.
The intervention may not be recognised within the medical establishment to be effective generally	*Examples:* Aromatherapy, reflexology, psychoanalytic psychotherapy for psychosis
The intervention may not be recognised within the medical establishment to be effective specifically for that patient with that disorder	*Example:* Acupuncture for psychotic symptoms
The intervention indicated is not accepted as needed by the patient	*Example:* Medication for psychotic symptoms; the patient's self-assessment may be very different to that of the professional or adverse effects are weighted more heavily by the patient than the professional in their assessment of risk/benefit
There is no effective medical intervention	*Example:* Possession states or religious faith is questioned
Treatment resistance	*Example:* Persistent psychotic symptoms
Intervention cannot be provided within the time scale requested	

should not be delivering these treatments if their efficacy is not proven. However, ethnic minority communities are demanding alternatives to pharmacological treatment (see Chapters 20 and 21). The scientific evaluation of such interventions is riddled with methodological difficulties (Ernst, 1995), especially concerning the selection of suitable placebo controls (Vincent & Lewith, 1995) and, for psychotherapies, suitable outcome measures. In the face of demand, social services may well fund the provision of alternative treatments where health services do not.

Change within any organisation is accompanied by ambivalence. If existing services are to adapt to the needs of ethnic minority patients, then practical steps should be taken immediately. Managerial priority is invariably given to ensuring that any new venture does not endanger existing working practices to the disadvantage of established service user groups, or that attempts to 'culturalise' a service do not place an unnecessary additional burden upon already busy clinical teams (Bhui *et al*, 1995*b*). One solution is that proposed by Dillard *et al* (1992), who described the development of 'focus teams' within each generic service. Each focus team is responsible for familiarisation with the community and allows the community to access their knowledge and skills. This model is not dissimilar to the link-worker model practised in New Zealand. Similar efforts are under way in the UK to ascertain the efficacy of providing link-workers who act as advocates as well as conduits of liaison between the community and the services. The advantage of the focus team is that the team, with different skill mixes, is responsible as a whole rather than one individual who may feel overwhelmed and isolated in the role of 'cultural representative' if not supported properly. The focus team should formally and informally gather information about the needs of the community and, regarding service delivery, facilitating strategic evolution of services and ways of avoiding fragmentation of services. They should ensure that the knowledge gathered is retained within the generic team irrespective of changes in staffing.

In-patient admission policies and procedures must be culturally sensitive if secondary care services are to be accepted by ethnic minority groups. Religious and cultural practices must be catered for and should include early involvement of religious leaders both in community and hospital settings. At a more practical level it may be a good idea for each service to indicate in their information packs how various needs of ethnic minorities (e.g. food, religion, women-only services) are being met.

Special issues in management of mental illness

In addition to community and secondary services, there are some specific issues that must be acknowledged in the management of mental illness among members of ethnic minorities.

Physical treatments

There is anecdotal and clinical evidence that, for some ethnic minorities at least, the use of higher doses of drugs and electro-convulsive therapy is more prevalent (Bhugra, 1993*b*; Bhui *et al*,

1995*a*). Although it has been suggested that people from southeast Asia and south Asia demonstrate clinical response at lower than average levels of neuroleptics, when compared with White Americans and Europeans, the data are often sketchy. There is no doubt that more pharmacological work needs to be done to deal with these very sensitive and pertinent issues. The use of such drugs and increased risks of side-effects make their acceptance very difficult. Similarly, sensitivity to alcohol and responses to antidepressant medication and anxiolytics have led some to suggest that each racial group may have unique psychodynamic and pharmacokinetic responses (Bhui *et al*, 1995*a*; Lin *et al*, 1995). However, a word of caution is needed here. The stress on individual racial and ethnic differences has historically lead to unfruitful, demeaning debates on biological superiority/inferiority of races; such debates further alienate and negate the cultural identity of ethnic minorities. However, a lack of exploration of genuine pharmacokinetic and pharmacodynamic differences may perpetuate the notion that complaints about medication from ethnic minority patients are unwarranted, and are then not heard.

The role of doctor–patient interaction in any consultation is vital (Bhugra 1993*a,b*). The use of medication as an alternative to a loss of autonomy and social control and unusual beliefs and behaviour are important grievances often ignored by clinicians.

Psychological therapies

The availability of psychological therapies across the country is patchy and the referral rates of patients from ethnic minorities are low. Several reasons have been put forward for this, including: perceived lack of use of psychological models in certain ethnic minorities; lack of demand for such services; lack of gender-specific therapists; and a perceived lack of culturally sensitive training in various psychotherapies. Psychotherapies available through the National Health Service have their roots in the West and tend to represent a Western ideal with emphasis on a nuclear family model; they may ignore or sometimes contradict the traditional beliefs and ideology of those with different value systems. As Littlewood (1992) emphasises:

> "...all societies make distinctions between desired and undesired states of being and have standardised forms of reconstructing experience, through the response of other people to return the individual to a state desired by the individual and community alike. At such level of abstraction, therapy is universal".

This is further confirmed by different types of culture-specific therapies developed in other cultures (Neki, 1975). In the UK the use of intercultural therapy and its success have been well documented by Kareem & Littlewood (1992; also see Lloyd & Bhugra, 1993; Bhugra & Bhui, 1998*b*). The quality of the relationship in psychotherapy sessions is more important than the ethnicity of therapists or their patients. It has been argued that in therapeutic encounters the exclusion of pain and hurt resulting from racism is resisted by the therapist, disguised under the notion of cultural sensitivity (Campling, 1989). There is evidence to suggest that group psychotherapy sessions in Urdu, Hindi or Punjabi can work with individuals (Bavington & Majid, 1986). Similarly, therapeutic community models of care have been used successfully, as have family intervention strategies with ethnic minority families. Families must be involved in regular meetings to discuss treatment options even if formal therapy sessions are not indicated. Such involvement has been shown to be particularly useful for the families of people from ethnic minorities with mental illness (Lin *et al*, 1991). An inbred reluctance on the part of the statutory services to involve families and to develop appropriate services to support carers often leaves ethnic minority patients unsettled and suspicious of the long-term intentions of social and health care service structures (see Box 4; also see Bhugra & Bhui, 1998*b*).

Cognitive therapy, according to MacCarthy (1987), is perhaps the most suitable therapy across ethnic minorities. Various techniques

---

Box 4
Psychotherapies

Establish the range of psychotherapies offered.
Ascertain at what stage assessment is offered.
Establish whether the therapy is offered as an alternative or in conjunction with drug therapies. Is there a review?
Involve patient in the decision.
Ascertain which diagnosis influences the choice of psychotherapy.
Establish which therapies are available to ethnic groups.
Find out whether multilingual therapies are available.
Establish which groups do not access these therapies. Why not?
Establish whether there is any training.
Find out about the existence of intercultural therapies.
Ask whether patients are satisfied.
Ascertain what the evaluative measures are.
Decide what the culturally appropriate outcomes are.
Establish whether interpreters or advocates are available.

such as verifying assumptions, generating alternative solutions and other strategies included in cognitive therapy can be extremely useful in working across cultures, as the acceptability of a range of behavioural options within social contexts can be explored as an integral form of therapy. Although many beliefs and values comprising cognitive sets are culturally determined, these can be readily understood if the therapist is prepared to listen with an open mind and by increasing the number of sessions necessary to achieve the same degree of understanding achieved with English-speaking British patients. Behavioural therapy has been said to be particularly well-adapted to cross-cultural work since it focuses on objectively observable and measurable phenomena (Bhugra, 1993*b*). However, attempts to modify sexual behaviour and social skills may prove to be more problematic.

Rehabilitation services

Rehabilitation with social skills assessment, assertiveness training and token economy may prove very difficult under certain circumstances. Deploying culture-affirming symbolism and encouraging identification with the patient's own cultural or religious group helps to nurture the ongoing development of cultural identity; usually this very identity has been fragmented and is under attack in a society which treats difference and skin colour as peculiar and threatening. Much of the distress faced by minorities is related to discrimination, disadvantage and loss of previous support structures including family and religious networks, homeland and a sense of belonging. Existing services may not allow the patients or their families positively to value their cultural and religious attributes which previously supported them and with which they identify. Appropriate local voluntary group contact and leisure activities should actively be encouraged (see Box 5).

Box 5
Rehabilitation

Cultural events should be incorporated in long-term care plans.
Special cooking, religious and spiritual needs should be acknowledged.
Differences in personal preferences for privacy in hospital should be taken
into account.
Establish which agencies are involved in long-term care.
Establish which skills are offered by the agencies.
Establish whether culturally positive events occur.
Employment and training opportunities should be provided.
Establish which core service components are available.

Box 6
Black women's health needs

Local initiatives for Black and other ethnic minority women.
Innovation in treatment approaches.
Evaluation of health needs.
Evaluation of cultural, religious and spiritual needs.
Evaluation of the level of patient satisfaction.
Ascertain the level of role satisfaction. Are they understood?
Decide whether any interventions are redundant.

Adopting a flexible approach to long-term care

Black women

Women's needs in relation to facilities in hospital and at home differ sufficiently for a separate assessment of their requirements to be made. There are different degrees and types of religious participation as well as degrees of privacy. The social significance of mental illness also differs for women and their traditional roles as carers may vary and contribute to further stress. Treatment packages which support a woman's role in family and society may positively encourage the continued, culturally appropriate application of mechanisms of resolving distress. Popular methods of child-rearing may not be assigned to women from other cultures and the impact of child separation and other life events is not the same across different ethnic communities. There is substantial need to involve Black women from different cultural and ethnic groups in discussing and developing appropriate levels and models of care (see Box 6).

Box 7
Evaluation of services

Ensure that local services are evaluated.
Ensure that ethnic groups are evaluated.
Are the evaluations carried out using specific methodologies?
How sensitive are the methods used?
How is access measured?
Routinely elicit views.
Consult with ethnic groups.
Provide information about services, take-up, hospital stay and success with
    services.
How is the community represented at various levels in various agencies?

Evaluation of new health and social care policy

The commissioner–provider split encourages a degree of account-ability in decision-making about service provision and evaluation with the NHS White Papers, and primary care grouping should make further innovation possible. New drugs, new psychological therapies and newer models of working are not being evaluated across cultural groups, except perhaps in pilot sites, which may make their duplication elsewhere difficult. Already alienated from existing services, the wave of new developments in services that are not evaluated can only result in further disadvantage to ethnic minority patients and their carers. Access to combined health and social care can be extremely complex, especially if language and customs inhibit successful completion of forms and other similar criteria required by the social and health care services.

Cultural sensitivity of new service structures should be evaluated. All schemes need to evaluate the impact of treatment modalities on Black people. The impact of court diversion, prison diversion, care management and the care programme approach, as well as a supervision register, needs to be studied for ethnic communities (see Box 7).

Staff and institutions

Each organisation should have an explicit policy on racism and harassment. Training in cross-cultural work is increasingly important. Health care workers must be involved in some sessional time devoted to Black organisations. This would form a very useful point of interactive contact between these organisations and health care services. This will allow a two-way education and will identify the role of voluntary organisations, lead to joint purchasing and allow a discussion of the research agenda and research findings.

Conclusions

We have only been able to address the most pertinent issues facing ethnic minority communities in Britain today. The issues of institutional and pervasive racism have to be borne in mind while planning services. There is much evidence to suggest that ethnic minorities suffer multiple disadvantages in gaining access to psychiatric services and, despite extensive restructuring and National Health Service reforms, attention to specific evaluations of services for ethnic minority patients has been minimal. The training of professionals at all levels within the services is a crucial factor. Voluntary organisations, in a true partnership with statutory services, can play a significant role in the development and provision of culturally appropriate services. The voluntary sector is suitably placed to act in patient advocacy roles and contribute to 'quality checks' of statutory services.

References

ADEBIMPE, V. (1994) Race, racism and epidemiological surveys. *Hospital and Community Psychiatry*, **45**, 27–31.

BAVINGTON, J. & MAJID, A. (1986) Psychiatric services for ethnic minority groups. In *Transcultural Psychiatry* (ed. J. L. Cox), pp 87–106. London: Croom Helm.

BENNETT, D. & FREEMAN, H. (1991) Principles and prospects. In *Community Psychiatry* (eds D. H. Bennett & H. Freeman), pp. 1–39. Edinburgh: Churchill Livingstone.

BHUGRA, D. (1993*a*) Influence of culture on presentation and management of patients. In *Principles of Social Psychiatry* (eds D. Bhugra & J. Leff), pp. 67–81, Oxford: Blackwell.

—— (1993*b*) Setting up services for ethnic minorities. In *Dimensions of Community Mental Health Care* (eds M. Weller & M. Muijen), pp. 116–134. London: W. B. Saunders.

——, BRIDGES, K. & THOMPSON, C. (1995) *Caring for a Community*, Council Report CR36. London: Royal College of Psychiatrists.

—— & BHUI, K. (1998*a*) Do problems persist in second generations? *Hospital Medicine*, **59**, 126–129.

—— & —— (1998*b*) Psychotherapy for ethnic minorities. *British Journal of Psychotherapy*, **14**, 310–326.

BHUI, K., CHRISTIE, Y. & BHUGRA, D. (1995*a*) The essential elements of culturally sensitive psychiatric services *International Journal of Social Psychiatry*, **41**, 242–256.

——, FOULDS, G., BAUBIN, F., *et al* (1995*b*) Developing culturally sensitive community services for the severely mentally ill: the PACT team's experience. *British Journal of Health Care*, **1**, 817–822.

CAMPLING, P. (1989) Race, culture and psychotherapy. *Psychiatric Bulletin*, **13**, 350–351.

DEPARTMENT OF HEALTH (1989) *Caring for People*. London: HMSO.

DILLARD, M., ANDONDIAN, L., FLORES, O., *et al* (1992) Culturally competent occupational therapy in a diversely populated mental health setting. *American Journal of Occupational Therapy*, **46**, 721–725.

ERNST, E. (1995) Complementary medicine: common misconceptions. *Journal of the Royal Society of Medicine*, **88**, 244–247.

GILLAM, S., JARMAN, B., WHITE, P. *et al* (1989) Ethnic differences in consultation rates in urban general practice. *British Medical Journal*, **289**, 953–957.

GOLDBERG, D. & HUXLEY, P. (1980) *Mental Illness in the Community*. London: Tavistock.

KAREEM, J. & LITTLEWOOD, R. (1992) *Intercultural Therapy: Themes, Interpretations and Practices*. Oxford: Blackwell Scientific.

LIN, K., MILLER, M., POLLARD, R., *et al* (1991) Ethnicity and family involvement in the treatment of schizophrenic patients. *Journal of Nervous and Mental Disease*, **179**, 631–633.

———, POLAND, R. & ANDERSON, D. (1995) Psychopharmacology, ethnicity & culture. *Transcultural Psychiatric Research Review*, **32**, 3–40.

LITTLEWOOD, R. (1992) How universal is something that we call psychotherapy? In *Intercultural Therapy. Themes, Interpretations and Practice* (eds J. Kareem & R. Littlewood), pp. 38–56. London: Blackwell Scientific.

LLOYD, K. (1993) Depression and anxiety among Afro-Caribbean general practice attenders in Britain. *International Journal of Social Psychiatry*, **39**, 1–9.

—— & BHUGRA, D. (1993) Cross-cultural aspects of psychotherapy. *International Review of Psychiatry*, **5**, 291–304.

MACCARTHY, B. (1987) Clinical work with ethnic minorities. In *New Developments in Clinical Psychology* (ed. F. N. Watts), pp. 122–139. Chichester: John Wiley.

NAZROO, J. (1997) *Ethnicity and Mental Health.* London: Policy Studies Institute.

NEKI, J. S. (1975) Psychotherapy in India: past, present and future. *American Journal of Psychotherapy*, **29**, 92–100.

SASHIDHARAN, S. (1993) Afro-Caribbeans and schizophrenia: the ethnic vulnerability hypothesis re-examined. *International Review of Psychiatry*, **5**, 129–144.

STRATHDEE, G. (1994) Psychiatry and general practice – a psychiatric perspective. In *Psychiatry and General Practice Today* (eds I. Pullen, G. Wilkinson, A. Wright & D. P. Gray), pp. 22–35. London: Royal College of Psychiatrists & Royal College of General Practioners.

—— & THORNICROFT, G. (1993) The principles of setting up mental health services in the community. In *Principles of Social Psychiatry* (eds D. Bhugra & J. Leff), pp. 473–489. Oxford: Blackwell.

VINCENT, C. & LEWITH, G. (1995) Placebo controls for acupuncture studies. *Journal of the Royal Society of Medicine*, **88**, 199–202.

23 The Fourth National Survey of Ethnic Minorities

SUNJAI GUPTA

Ethnic minorities comprise approximately 6% of the total population of Great Britain (Haskey, 1996). Of these, just under half are from the Indian subcontinent, nearly one-third are African–Caribbean and 4% are Chinese in origin.

This chapter summarises some of the evidence for differences in mental health between members of Black and ethnic minority groups and the White population (though some important groups, such as the Irish, have not been covered; Bracken *et al*, 1998). In particular it focuses on new data from the Fourth National Survey of Ethnic Minorities – the importance of which is highlighted by the fact that there are comparatively few national sources in this area. I aim to show that the Survey potentially provides a way to clarify a number of issues arising out of previous studies, but will also argue that it leaves unanswered several questions that can only be resolved by further research.

Mortality

A recently published document (Department of Health, 1996*a*) makes clear that the burden due to a given illness may be considered at a number of different levels, the first of which is mortality. In the case of mental illness the most conspicuous form of this is, of course, suicide, and Raleigh (1996) has analysed data on suicide and undetermined injury for England and Wales for 1988–1992 and 1979–1983[1]. In 1988–1992 the age-standardised mortality ratio (SMR) from suicide in men born on the Indian subcontinent was significantly lower than the national average. Suicide ratios were also significantly low in men born in Bangladesh, Sri Lanka and Pakistan.

However, there was a statistically significant excess (43%) of suicide in Indian women. East African-born women also showed an excess, of 54% over the national ratio. Raleigh argues that the international literature consistently shows higher rates of suicide in young south Asian women, whereas lower rates are found in Black Americans and in the Caribbean population (see Chapter 12).

These data are a cause for concern even though in absolute terms the numbers of deaths involved are comparatively small. Furthermore, psychological factors may play a role in mortality from other conditions as well. For example, Wild & McKeigue (1997) report that SMRs for coronary heart disease were highest for south Asian men and women and east African men. In their study SMRs for cerebrovascular disease (stroke) were also significantly higher than the national average for nearly all immigrant groups in 1989–1992, except those born in east Africa, the highest ratios being for west African immigrants.

McKeigue & Sevak (1994) conclude that:

> "The most plausible explanation for the high rates of coronary heart disease in south Asians is that a pattern of metabolic disturbances associated with insulin resistance and central obesity underlies the high rates of both coronary heart disease and diabetes".

However, Wild & McKeigue (1997) point out that Afro-Caribbean people have comparatively low rates of coronary heart disease in spite of their high prevalence of diabetes and hypertension. This suggests that factors other than insulin resistance may play a part in the high rates of coronary heart disease in people from south Asia. Shaukat & Cruickshank (1993) refer to data from India showing that patients with myocardial infarction had not only increased type A behaviours but also increased levels of anxiety and depression. They argue that in these groups, in Britain, type A behaviour may not present typically but minor psychiatric symptoms may be exhibited instead.

Fredrikson (1986) reviewed evidence which suggested that while Black subjects may have enhanced vascular reactivity to external stimuli, they may show lower heart rate reactivity. Furthermore,

---

1. Ethnic origin is not recorded on death certificates and as a result analyses of mortality cannot be carried out by ethnicity, only by country of birth. As a result second-generation members of ethnic minority groups (who form an ever increasing proportion) who were born in this country cannot be identified separately and are included with the indigenous population. Similarly, those of British origin who were born abroad are included with the foreign-born population.

he argues that this may help to explain why they have high rates of mortality from hypertension and stroke, but low mortality from coronary heart disease. Data in this area are conflicting, but it is interesting that Sayer *et al* (1997) demonstrated an absence of the normal circadian and seasonal rhythms in myocardial infarction in people from south Asia, and this supports the view that there may be ethnic differences in autonomic function which may interact with external stressors to influence patterns of cardiovascular disease.

Morbidity

Secondary care

Mortality, of course, represents only the 'tip of the iceberg' of burden due to mental ill-health. The next level is that of secondary care, and there is evidence again for differences between ethnic groups (see Chapters 5 and 19). For example, Cochrane & Bal (1989) analysed admissions to mental hospitals in England in 1981 and found that the people born outside the UK tended to have higher rates of admission for schizophrenia than the native-born population. Since then, local studies have suggested that schizophrenia may be diagnosed in Afro-Caribbean people approximately 3–6 times more often than in White people (Department of Health, 1996*b*).

More recent studies suggest that the differential may be either lower (Bhugra *et al,* 1997) or higher (Harrison *et al,* 1997) than this. Harrison *et al* also showed that the excess applied to all psychotic disorders, not only schizophrenia. Bhugra *et al* found that unemployment was related to the outcome of schizophrenia but this effect disappeared when ethnicity was allowed for. South Asian rates were higher than in White people in those over 30 years old, and lower than the Caribbean rates except in women older than 30 (among whom they were higher).

Gupta (1993) has suggested that the overall pattern of schizophrenia in ethnic minority groups is best explained by an interaction between constitutional and environmental factors. However, it is worth considering the implications of the 'pathways to care' model described by Goldberg & Huxley (1980)and the possibility that the permeability of the 'filters' which regulate movement between the different levels of care may vary between different subgroups in the population. For example, it has been argued (Sashidharan & Francis, 1993) that the apparently high rates of schizophrenia in African–Caribbean people might be due in part to their pattern of interaction with services.

This suspicion has been fuelled by other evidence of differential service use. Lipsedge (1993), for example, reviewed data which suggested that Black patients may be more likely to be admitted compulsorily (see also Davies *et al*, 1996), more likely to receive high-dose neuroleptic therapy when disturbed, and more likely to drop-out of rehabilitation and after-care programmes. South Asian people may be prescribed antidepressants in lower doses, but may be more likely than White people to receive electroconvulsive therapy. Gupta (1991*a*, 1992) has shown that south Asian patients were less likely to be readmitted but also more likely to be lost to follow-up.

Primary care

Morbidity statistics from general practice (McCormick *et al*, 1993) show that for both males and females a higher proportion of White than Indian people consulted their general practitioner (GP) for mental disorders. However, a survey of mental health provision in Newham showed that, while Asians were under-represented among those being given mental health care in the National Health Service, they were more likely to be found among the service users of voluntary agencies that accepted either self-referrals or offered a specific service to the Asian community (Gupta, 1990).

After adjusting for socio-demographic variables there was a general tendency in the morbidity statistics for fewer Black people to consult (especially Black female children) except among the elderly: Black elderly men were significantly more likely to consult. However, Boneham *et al* (1997) studied elderly members of ethnic minorities in Liverpool who were suffering from depression and dementia, and found that despite high levels of physical and mental impairment, levels of contact with services and support were not correspondingly high. For example, 87% had visited their GP in the past year, but only 35% had actually talked about psychological symptoms (see Chapter 11).

Rait *et al* (1996) have also argued that ethnic elders suffering from mental illnesses may be a particularly vulnerable group, and have suggested the use of culturally appropriate screening instruments to aid recognition. Evidence for the value of screening in the general population is conflicting (Johnstone & Goldberg, 1976; Hoeper *et al*, 1984) but studies in the USA have shown that screening in general medical settings may improve the detection rate in groups among whom this rate is low (including Black subjects; Shapiro *et al*, 1987) and may also be particularly helpful in those who present with a high proportion of somatic symptoms (Magruder-Habib *et al*, 1990).

This may be particularly relevant for members of ethnic minorities. For example, Wilson & MacCarthy (1994) have shown in London that among those who exceeded the threshold for a possible psychiatric disorder as assessed by a screening questionnaire, south Asian patients were more likely than native English patients to say that they had consulted their GP for a physical problem alone, and the south Asian people were less likely to be diagnosed as having a psychiatric disorder. Commander *et al* (1997*a,b*) also found in Birmingham that case recognition by GPs was higher in White than in Black or south Asian people. Such findings have important implications for services both in this country and elsewhere (Gupta, 1991*b*; Sartorius, 1997).

Community studies: the Fourth National Survey of Ethnic Minorities

As we have seen, suicide represents a small, though important, fraction of the total burden due to mental illness. Many studies of schizophrenia in African–Caribbean people (though not all) are potentially open to the criticism that they reflect the pattern of interaction with secondary care services resulting in different conspicuous rather than actual rates. On the other hand, studies in primary care have led to concern that the reservoir of hidden 'minor' mental morbidity in the population may also be disproportionately large in members of ethnic minorities. However, early attempts to test this directly, using surveys, appeared to point in a different direction and contributed to the impression that rates of mental illness in south Asian people, for example, were similar to or lower than those of the indigenous population (Department of Health, 1992).

Ideally, these issues should be resolved through national community studies. The findings of the recent National Psychiatric Morbidity Study (Meltzer *et al*, 1995) were, however, difficult to interpret because of the small numbers in the sample who regarded themselves as belonging to minority ethnic groups. Despite this, compared with White women, depression was twice as prevalent in West Indian and African women as in White women and this reinforced the need for a larger study focusing specifically on ethnicity.

An example is the Fourth National Survey of Ethnic Minorities (Nazroo, 1997, 1998) which was carried out in 1993–1994 and was a representative study in England and Wales, covering groups which included Caribbean, Indian, African–Asian, Pakistani, Bangladeshi and Chinese people. It was the first comprehensive study of ethnic differences in the rates of mental illness that was based on detection rather than treatment rates or suicide. Interviews were carried out by ethnically-matched interviewers in the language(s) of the respondents' choice. Parts of the revised version of the Clinical Interview Schedule (CIS–R; Lewis *et al*, 1992) were used to identify people with possible depression, and the Psychosis Screening Questionnaire (Bebbington & Nayani, 1995) was used to identify those with a possible psychotic illness. A proportion of those who scored positively on either of these instruments were followed up and underwent an interview based on the Present State Examination (version nine; Wing *et al*, 1974).

Full accounts of the methodology and data derived from the Survey are presented elsewhere (Nazroo, 1997, 1998), but some salient findings are reviewed here. In line with the National Psychiatric Morbidity Survey, the Fourth National Survey found that Caribbean people had higher rates of depression than White people. However, they were far less likely than White people to receive treatment for it. Surprisingly, in view of the data on suicide presented earlier, women in the south Asian groups did not have a higher rate than White women of reported suicidal thoughts. Furthermore, the Survey found that rates of mental illness among south Asian people were apparently low.

However, this was not true of those who were born in Britain, those who migrated under the age of 11 years or who were fluent in English. Furthermore, there was evidence that the initial interview was less reliable for the south Asian group, and that the Western measures of mental illness did not work well for them. For example there were difficulties in translating the term 'depression' into south Asian languages(Leff has also suggested this; see Chapter 5). Interestingly, those south Asian respondents who did score above a threshold on the depression scale of the CIS–R were less likely than their White counterparts to be taking antidepressants or minor tranquillisers, though those who scored above a threshold on the psychosis screening questionnaire were more likely to be taking major tranquillisers.

One particularly unexpected finding was the fact that the rate of schizophrenia for Caribbean people was less than twice that of White people, and for Caribbean men the rate was very similar. However, these data refer to the prevalence of illness at the time of interview. There is evidence that schizophrenia may have a better prognosis in Caribbean than in White people (McKenzie *et al*, 1995), and this (and other methodological factors) may help to explain these surprising findings (Nazroo, 1997, 1998).

Also of interest are the findings of the Survey regarding the relationship between social position and the risk of mental illness. Among the Caribbean group those in households without a full-time worker had the highest rate of psychosis, but those in households with a manually employed worker appeared to have lower rates than those in households with a non-manual worker, and most of the differences between the Caribbean and the White groups could be accounted for by the high rate in these latter Caribbean households.

In terms of neurotic disorder, for Caribbean, Indian/African–Asian and White people there was a reasonably clear relationship: those in non-manual households had the best health and those in households without a full-time worker had the worst health, though there was no difference between the manual and non-manual categories for the Caribbean group and depression. For the Pakistani/Bangladeshi group there did not appear to be a clear relationship between socio-economic status and neurotic disorder. Furthermore, the Bangladeshi group, despite being worse off economically than the Indian/African–Asian group, had a lower rate of mental illness.

This finding in particular bears scrutiny in view of evidence from other data collected as part of the Fourth National Survey and other studies. The Survey showed that, compared to White people, Pakistani and Bangladeshi people were 50% more likely to have described their health as 'fair' or 'poor'. The Health Education Authority's Black and Minority Ethnic Groups in England Survey (Health Education Authority, 1995) also showed that the single most frequently mentioned health risk by any of the different groups was the effect of poor housing, which was identified by the Bangladeshi community. Finally, MacCarthy & Craissati (1989) found that Bangladeshi people reported more serious life events and chronic difficulties, and correspondingly more symptoms of psychological disturbance, than their indigenous neighbours. Given these facts, the comparatively low rates of mental illness found among Bangladeshi people in the Fourth National Survey are particularly surprising.

Conclusion

In general, the Fourth National Survey represents a major advance on previous work on mental health in ethnic minorities. Nevertheless, it leaves a number of unanswered questions. For example, Nazroo (1998) acknowledges that Western assessments of mental illness may have failed adequately to identify mental distress in Asian people. One possible explanation is that symptom groups from the CIS–R covering somatic symptoms were specifically excluded. However, a recent World Health Organization study failed to detect any trend for somatisation disorder to be more or less common in 'developing' compared with 'developed' countries (Gureje *et al*, 1997). Similarly, in India, Patel *et al* (1998) found that the General Health Questionnaire (GHQ–12; Goldberg & Williams, 1988) and a screening instrument based on somatic symptoms were both equally effective in picking up psychiatric illness as assessed by patients and care providers.

Depending on the outcome of the pilot studies, the GHQ is likely to be used in the 1999 Health Survey for England (Gupta, 1994) which will focus on ethnic minorities. This will provide additional information about the mental health of these groups and about its relationship to physical health as assessed by both subjective and objective measures. Such developments are complementary to the independent inquiry into health inequalities which is being chaired by Sir Donald Acheson. They are also in line with the government's new health strategy which stresses the importance of such inequalities (including those between different ethnic groups) and which proposes mental illness as a priority area for future action (Department of Health, 1998).

References

BEBBINGTON, P. & NAYANI, T. (1995) The Psychosis Screening Questionnaire. *International Journal of Methods in Psyhiatric Research*, **5**, 11–19.

BHUGRA, D., LEFF, J. & MALLETT, R., *et al* (1997) Incidence and outcome of schizophrenia in Whites, African–Caribbeans and Asians in London. *Psychological Medicine*, **27**, 791–798.

BONEHAM, M. A., WILLIAMS, K. E. & COPELAND, J. R. M. (1997) Elderly people from ethnic minorities in Liverpool: mental illness, unmet need and barriers to service use. *Health and Social Care in the Community*, **5**, 173–180.

BRACKEN, P. J., GREENSLADE, L., GRIFFIN, B., *et al* (1998) Mental health and ethnicity: an Irish dimension. *British Journal of Psychiatry*, **172**, 103–105.

COCHRANE, R. & BAL, S. S. (1989) Mental hospital admission rates of immigrants to England: a comparison of 1971 and 1981. *Social Psychiatry and Psychiatric Epidemiology*, **24**, 2–11.

COMMANDER, M. J., SASHIDHARAN, S. P., ODELL, S. M., *et al* (1997*a*) Access to mental health care in an inner-city health district. I: Pathways into and within specialist psychiatric services. *British Journal of Psychiatry*, **170**, 312–316.

——, ——, ——, *et al* (1997*b*) Access to mental health care in an inner-city health district. II: Association with demographic factors. *British Journal of Psychiatry*, **170**, 317–320.

DAVIES, S., THORNICROFT, G. & LEESE, M., *et al* (1996) Ethnic differences in risk of compulsory psychiatric admission among representative cases of psychosis in London. *British Medical Journal*, **312**, 533–537.

DEPARTMENT OF HEALTH (1992) *On the State of the Public Health 1991*. London: HMSO.

—— (1996*a*) *Burdens of Disease. A Discussion Document*. Leeds: NHS Executive.

—— (1996*b*) *On the State of the Public Health 1995*. London: HMSO.

— (1998) *Our Healthier Nation. A Contract for Health. A Consultation Paper.* London: HMSO.

FREDRIKSON, M. (1986) Racial differences in cardiovascular reactivity to mental stress in essential hypertension. *Journal of Hypertension,* **4**, 325–331.

GOLDBERG, D. P. & HUXLEY, P. (1980) *Mental Illness in the Community.* London: Tavistock.

—— & WILLIAMS, P. (1988) *A User's Guide to the General Health Questionnaire.* Windsor: NFER–Nelson.

GUPTA, S. (1990) The mental health of Asians in Britain (letter). *British Medical Journal,* **301**, 240.

— (1991*a*) Psychosis in migrants from the Indian subcontinent and English-born controls. A preliminary study on the use of psychiatric services. *British Journal of Psychiatry,* **159**, 222–225.

— (1991*b*) *The Mental Health Problems of Migrants. A Report from Six European Countries.* Copenhagen: WHO Regional Office for Europe.

— (1992) Psychosis in Asian immigrants from the Indian subcontinent: preliminary findings from a follow-up study including a survey of general practitioners. *Social Psychiatry and Psychiatric Epidemiology,* **27**, 242–244.

— (1993) Can environmental factors explain the epidemiology of schizophrenia in immigrant groups? *Social Psychiatry and Psychiatric Epidemiology,* **28**, 263–266.

— (1994) Health surveys as a tool for government: the Health Survey for England as a paradigm case. *Archives in Public Health,* **52**, 99–113.

GUREJE, O., SIMON, G. E., USTUN, T. B., *et al* (1997) Somatization in cross-cultural perspective: a World Health Organization study in primary care. *American Journal of Psychiatry,* **154**, 989–995.

HARRISON, G., GLAZEBROOK, C. & BREWIN, J. (1997) Increased incidence of psychotic disorders in immigrants from the Caribbean to the United Kingdom. *Psychological Medicine,* **27**, 799–806.

HASKEY, J. (1996) The ethnic minority populations resident in private households – estimates by country and metropolitan districts of England and Wales. *Population Trends,* **63**, 22–35.

HEALTH EDUCATION AUTHORITY (1995) *Black and Minority Ethnic Groups in England.* London: Health Education Authority.

HOEPER, E. W., NYCZ, G. R., KESSLER, L. G., *et al* (1984) The usefulness of screening for mental illness. *Lancet, i*, 33–35.

JOHNSTONE, A. & GOLDBERG, D. (1976) Psychiatric screening in general practice. A controlled trial. *Lancet, i*, 605–608.

LEWIS, G., PELOSI, A. J. ARAYA, R., *et al* (1992) Measuring psychiatric disorder in the community: a standardized assessment for use by lay interviewers. *Psychological Medicine,* **22**, 465–486.

LIPSEDGE, M. (1993) Mental health: access to care for Black and ethnic minority people. In *Access to Health Care for People from Black and Ethnic Minorities* (eds A. Hopkins & V. Bahl), pp. 169–185. London: Royal College of Physicians.

MCCORMICK, A., FLEMING, D. & CHARLTON, J. (1993) *Morbidity Statistics from General Practice. Fourth National Study 1991–1992.* London: HMSO.

MCKEIGUE, P. & SEVAK, L. (1994) *Coronary Heart Disease in South Asian Communities.* London: Health Education Authority.

MCKENZIE, K., VAN OS, J., FAHY, T., *et al* (1995) Psychosis with good prognosis in Afro-Caribbean people now living in the United Kingdom. *British Medical Journal,* **311**, 1325–1328.

MACCARTHY, B. & CRAISSATI, J. (1989) Ethnic differences in response to adversity: a community sample of Bangladeshis and their indigenous neighbours. *Social Psychiatry and Psychiatric Epidemiology,* **24**, 196–201.

MAGRUDER-HABIB, K., ZUNG, W. K. & FEUSSNER, J. R. (1990) Improving physicians' recognition and treatment of depression in general medical care. Results from a randomized clinical trial. *Medical Care,* **28**, 239–250.

254   *Gupta*

MELTZER, H., GILL, B., PETTICREW, M., *et al* (1995) *The Prevalence of Psychiatric Morbidity Among Adults Living in Private Households.* London: HMSO.

NAZROO, J. Y. (1997) *Ethnicity and Mental Health.* London: Policy Studies Institute.

—— (1998) Rethinking the relationship between ethnicity and mental health: the British Fourth National Survey of Ethnic Minorities. *Social Psychiatry and Psychiatric Epidemiology,* **33**, 145–148.

PATEL, V., PEREIRA, J. & MANN, A. H. (1998) Somatic and psychological models of common mental disorder in primary care in India. *Psychological Medicine,* **28**, 135–143.

RAIT, G., BURNS, A., CHEW, C., *et al* (1996) Age, ethnicity and mental illness, a triple whammy. *British Medical Journal,* **313**, 1347–1344.

RALEIGH, V. S. (1996) Suicide patterns and trends in people of Indian subcontinent and Caribbean origin in England and Wales. *Ethnicity and Health,* **1**, 55–63.

SARTORIUS, N. (1997) Psychiatry in the framework of primary health care: a threat or boost to psychiatry? *American Journal of Psychiatry,* **154**, 67–72.

SASHIDHARAN, S. P. & FRANCIS, E. (1993) Epidemiology, ethnicity and schizophrenia. In *"Race" and Health in Contemporary Britain* (ed. W. I. U. Ahmad), pp. 96–113. Open University Press.

SAYER, J. W., WILKINSON, P., RANJADAYALAN, K., *et al* (1997) Attenuation or absence of circadian and seasonal rhythms of acute myocardial infarction. *Heart,* **77**, 325–329.

SHAPIRO, S., GERMAN, P. S., SKINNER, E. A. , *et al* (1987) An experiment to change detection and management of mental morbidity in primary care. *Medical Care,* **25**, 327–339.

SHAUKAT, N. & CRUICKSHANK, J. K. (1993) Coronary artery disease: impact on Black and ethnic minority people. In *Access to Health Care for People from Black and Ethnic Minorities* (eds A. Hopkins & V. Bahl), pp. 133–146. London: Royal College of Physicians.

WILD, S. & McKEIGUE, P. (1997) Cross-sectional analysis of mortality by country of birth in England and Wales, 1970–92. *British Medical Journal,* **314**, 705–708.

WILSON, M. & MACCARTHY, B. (1994) GP consultation as a factor in the low rate of mental health services use by Asians. *Psychological Medicine,* **24**, 113–119.

WING, J. K., COOPER, J. E. & SARTORIUS, N. (1974) *Measurement and Classification of Psychiatric Symptoms: An Instruction Manual for the PSE and Catego Program.* Cambridge: Cambridge University Press.

24   Conclusions

DINESH BHUGRA and VEENA BAHL

Ethnicity and the practice of cross-cultural psychiatry are at a crossroads. It is evident from Gray (Chapter 20) and Gluckman's cautions (Chapter 17) that clinical as well as academic psychiatry have received bad press in this country. This volume has attempted to move the agenda forward to improve the health of ethnic minority groups. There is evidence that psychiatric and psychological morbidity in ethnic minory groups are fairly extensive and vary across different groups, yet the use of services by people from the ethnic minorities is poor.

This may reflect the rigidity of statutory services or retention and use of different explanatory models by members of ethnic minorities. It may also reflect a genuine need for alternatives that are offered by voluntary organisations who may not be as inflexible and bureaucratically bound. One of the advantages of the National Health Service changes is that commissioners can pick and choose the kind of services they wish. With the publication of NHS White Papers and a Green Paper the agenda of mental health has moved forward and those of minority ethnic groups have become more prominent.

Training of professionals

One of the primary aims for service providers is the adequate, appropriate and successful training of their employees. Training should include issues such as cultural sensitivity, as well as a whole way of thinking, and should involve discussion of alternative models of spirituality and treatments that are available and what can be expected. For medical and nursing staff this training has to start at the basic undergraduate level. The training may involve social scientists, users of the services and voluntary organisations as well as other agencies who can provide essential background, models of care and knowledge of appropriate pathways into care. For other members of the multi-disciplinary teams such training, especially in local catchment areas, is vital. Ongoing training and continuing professional development are important requirements in the field of cross-cultural psychiatry.

The future

Clinical agenda

With emphasis on care in the community it is vital that purchasers and providers work with target communities in their catchment areas to identify the communities' needs. There is movement towards health services which are led by primary care. Therefore, general practitioners (GPs) are to be involved in this task. There is anecdotal and research evidence that some communities do not use primary care because they feel that GPs are not sensitive to their needs, or that GPs follow medical models which the patients and their carers find completely inappropriate. Although some communities may seek help from voluntary organisations, this too is not universal, partly because patients and their carers may see this as a second-class service and partly because they are worried about confidentiality. Thus, one model would be for the statutory services, primary and secondary care services and the community mental health care team to work closely with voluntary organisations in order to understand models of explanation and models of acceptable care, and to provide services which are user-friendly, appropriately funded and culturally and socially accessible and appropriate (Bhugra *et al*, 1995). More work needs to be done to develop services which rely on patients' needs rather than clinical diagnoses, as at the moment services focus too strictly on psychopathology and symptoms. This would allow patients and their carers to express their requirements and to accept help. Clinical services must be used not only for curative purposes, but also for preventative strategies by developing public health models. This can be achieved through work with communities, in schools, offices and places of work, towards education about the prevention of mental ill health, treatment methods and processes which can be used by those who need it. Ethnic monitoring will allow the planners to obtain an accurate picture of the needs and numbers involved.

Research agenda

Research on ethnic minorities' needs and psychological morbidity must involve the communities themselves. This is vital if the research is to establish the true levels of morbidity and to understand the interpretation of these results in full consultation with the community.

Hopefully, the period of 'looking in from outside' is over. The leaders as well as the members of communities must be involved in identifying the research questions most pertinent to their needs. The role of 'cultural broker' in such circumstances could prove to be a useful concept. Researchers must also take responsibility for the implementation of their findings, which must be appropriate and useful for the provision of services. Thus, the role of purchasers and providers in the discussion of research and its processes must be clear from the very beginning.

Newer models

Gluckman (Chapter 17) has identified some innovative projects for providing services for ethnic minorities. It is crucial that the people involved in these services are not seen as 'outsiders'. The providers must be able to incorporate innovative and useful ideas which will contribute to and make significant changes in the provision of services that are acceptable to the community. Services involving voluntary organisations, primary and secondary care and other agencies in the community must be developed, funded and resourced jointly, with each component having an equally valid say in their running, thereby ensuring the acceptance and success of such services. The recent NHS White Papers and Green Paper offer a welcome initiative.

Conclusions

Ethnicity forms only one, significant, part of any individual. Their religious, spiritual and psychological needs have to be balanced with the historical context of their arrival and growth in the UK, without ignoring the individual's physical needs. It would be ideal if the communities themselves were able to generate research questions which could be investigated by researchers who have a stake in the projects. Encouraging a community to work with researchers in the interpretation of results could help to minimise mistakes. Effective implementation of these research findings would facilitate the provision of adequate, culturally sensitive services.

Reference

BHUGRA, D., BRIDGES, K. & THOMPSON, C. (1995) *Caring for a Community*, Council Report CR36. London: Royal College of Psychiatrists.

Index

Compiled by LINDA M. ENGLISH